When Communities Assess Their AIDS Epidemics

When Communities Assess Their AIDS Epidemics

Results of Rapid Assessment of HIV/AIDS in Eleven U.S. Cities

Benjamin P. Bowser, Ernest Quimby, and Merrill Singer

LEXINGTON BOOKS

A division of
ROWMAN & LITTLEFIELD PUBLISHERS, INC.
Lanham • Boulder • New York • Toronto • Plymouth, UK

LEXINGTON BOOKS

A division of Rowman & Littlefield Publishers, Inc.
A wholly owned subsidiary of The Rowman & Littlefield Publishing Group, Inc.
4501 Forbes Boulevard, Suite 200
Lanham, MD 20706

Estover Road
Plymouth PL6 7PY
United Kingdom

British Library Cataloguing in Publication Information Available

Library of Congress Cataloging-in-Publication Data

When communities assess their AIDS epidemics : results of rapid assessment of HIV/AIDS in eleven U.S. cities / [edited by] Benjamin P. Bowser, Ernest Quimby, and Merrill Singer.
p. ; cm.
Includes bibliographical references and index.
ISBN-13: 978-0-7391-0752-2 (cloth : alk. paper)
ISBN-10: 0-7391-0752-6 (cloth : alk. paper)
1. AIDS (Disease)—United States. 2. HIV infections—United States. 3. Cities and towns—United States. I. Bowser, Benjamin P. II. Quimby, Ernest. III. Singer, Merrill.
[DNLM: 1. Acquired Immunodeficiency Syndrome—epidemiology—United States. 2. Acquired Immunodeficiency Syndrome—prevention & control—United States. 3. African Americans—United States. 4. Community Networks—United States. 5. Organizational Case Studies—United States. 6. Risk Assessment—United States. WC 503.4 AA1 W567 2007]
RA643.83.W4545 2007
614.5'99392—dc22 2006102794

Printed in the United States of America

™ The paper used in this publication meets the minimum requirements of American National Standard for Information Sciences—Permanence of Paper for Printed Library Materials, ANSI/NISO Z39.48–1992.

Contents

Preface

Eric Goosby, M.D.

The HIV/AIDS epidemic continues to impact communities throughout the world. It occurs within social, political and economic contexts described in this book.

UNAIDS/WHO estimates 40 million adults and children worldwide are living with HIV in 2005. The United States comprises 1.2 million, Western Europe 720,000, East Asia 870,000, South East Asia 7.4 million, and the largest numbers continue to be in Sub-Saharan Africa at 25.8 million. The epidemic in the United States continues to increase in both the number of new annual HIV seroconversions and, through advances in treatment, the number of people progressing in their HIV infection to a diagnosis of AIDS. Both the new seroconversions and the new AIDS diagnoses are predominantly occurring in men who have sex with men (63%); however, in women the transmission is predominantly through heterosexual contact (80%).

The racial impact disproportionately affects African Americans, who make up 12% of the United States census, now making up over 45% of the cumulative AIDS cases overall. Looking at more recent trends in the past ten years, we see African American rates of AIDS cases diagnosed was greater than ten times the rate for whites and almost three times the rate for Hispanics. AIDS was diagnosed for African American women at a rate greater than twenty-five times the rate for white women. The rate of AIDS diagnosed for African American men was 8 times the rate for white men (CDC 2003 data). Since the first reported HIV/AIDS in children less than thirteen years of age, African American children have made up greater than 90% of the cases. Most disturbing is the recently published data looking at HIV prevalence rates in five major cities in the United States showing up to a 48% sero-prevalence rate in some communities of African American men who have sex with men. Finally, injection drug use (IDU) has directly or indirectly accounted for more than 36% of the cumulative AIDS cases in the United States. IDU-associated AIDS accounts for a larger proportion of cases among women than among men. Since the epidemic began in 1981, more than 58% of all AIDS cases among women have been attributed to injection drug use or sex with partners who inject drugs, compared with 30% of cases among men. Non-injection drug use such as crack cocaine, powder cocaine and alcohol, contribute to the spread of the epidemic when users trade sex for drugs or money or when they engage in risky sexual behaviors that they might not engage in when sober.

The advent of effective antiretroviral agents, first discovered in the mid-80s with zidovudine (AZT), has lead to dramatic effects on the natural history of HIV. The frequency and severity of opportunistic infections have dramatically decreased morbidity and mortality seen in AIDS patients. Mono therapy led to dual therapy in the late 1980s and early 1990s with other nucleoside reverse transcriptase inhibitors and the discovery of the more potent protease inhibitors in 1994, which continue to evolve to the present.

Progress continued with the identification of the non-nucleoside reverse transcriptase inhibitors and the newer fusion inhibitor. Our ability to either prevent opportunistic infections with prophylaxis or treat it once acquired has lessened the frequency of infections and decreased deaths dramatically. These therapeutic advances changed the natural history of the infection in individuals by slowing progression (drop in viral load) and improving immune function (immune restoration, rise in CD4 lymphocytes). In all cohorts being followed, the number of AIDS deaths has continued to decrease each year for those on therapy.

People in treatment have stabilized their physical declines and in most instances returned to a much higher overall level of function. It has allowed HIV+ people to perceive themselves as continuing into the future and thereby regaining some control of their own self-perceptions. The movement from high risk behavior, to exposure, to infection and death has been partially corrected for those individuals who are entered and retained in medical care.

The tragedy of continued HIV expansion and its disproportionate impact on communities of color and women will not be altered until we acknowledge that the HIV epidemic is made up of multiple, separate micro-epidemics in any given city or region of our country. Each of these micro-epidemics has its own population, and its own motivators that inform behavior patterns and define specific access conduits to medical and social services. These conduits may or may not be utilized by the high risk populations due to a variety of real and perceived barriers. Our ability to stop the expanding edge of this epidemic is to understand how to respond to the factors that increase or decrease access and retention in medical care. The challenge to the public health system, at local, state and national levels, is to define what the barriers to care are, especially as perceived by the impacted populations, and to take this knowledge and let it inform how we design our medical delivery systems and target our prevention interventions.

Our public health departments have not developed enough effective programs that allow these high risk communities making up their HIV epidemic to be embraced in a continuum of medical care and services for the duration of their lives. Public health department activities are often overshadowed by police department strategies due to the under prioritization of public health and social service programs by local governments.

We will not be effective at ending the dual epidemics of illicit drug use and the HIV epidemic until we begin to see the active drug user not just as a felon, but also as a patient burdened by a disease—a disease that has been shown to respond to the convergence of social services, drug treatment and comprehensive medical services.

Our society has supported multiple strategies responding to the needs of these largely disenfranchised populations. Law enforcement has dominated the response. Public health measures have required a motivated patient to gain access to care and treatment and as a result have not made durable inroads into interfacing our prevention/treatment programs with high risk populations. We will not be successful in stopping the chronic movement of HIV into high risk communities and the general population until we admit that our current strategies are only marginally effective.

This book describes multiple attempts by departments of health and members of civil society to develop qualitative methodologies that allows for a "dialogue" between public health decision makers and the impacted micro-epidemic population. The dialogue is for the expressed purpose of taking the information and using it to develop unique strategies to better interface medical, social and drug treatment services with each micro-epidemic population. Most of the examples given in the book identified strategies that would be effective for specific communities in specific geographic locations and not broad "city-wide" programs that variably apply to all high risk groups. The use of geo-mapping, targeted interviews carried out by those trusted by the targeted community, focus groups and skilled analysis, are some of the ingredients that will enhance our ability to effectively respond to the HIV/AIDS epidemic in the United States.

The unmeasured burden of human loss will never be accurately defined, but what is clear is that it has impacted us as individuals and as societies in ways that we have just begun to appreciate. The epidemic is not over. It has continued to impact men who have sex with men (MSMs) and injection drug users, and has anchored itself in women, especially African American women. This disproportionate impact attributable to injection drug use has been observed for over a decade. Strategies that incorporate aggressive tools to identify clandestine high risk pockets of behavior in our inner cities and rural areas are critical to our success. The RARE qualitative methodology is such a tool. I hope this book triggers a new commitment by departments of health at all levels to see their role as including the development of multiple unique strategies to position the public health response directly in front of the conduits through which the HIV virus continues to expand into our communities. The ability to engage communities in effective, trusted dialogue over long periods of time is facilitated by RARE methodologies and defines a new relevance to the role public health departments must play in improving the health of individuals and groups.

The contributors do much more than provide appropriate and useful statistical overviews of the epidemic. An emphasis is placed on public policy, not merely methodologies. The editors' commendable efforts are ultimately aimed at effecting public policy, not merely promoting academic discourse. You will find these chapters to be sobering and windows on the epidemic of our times.

January 17, 2006

Introduction

Louis Kushnick
Ahmed Iqbal Ullah Race Relations Resource Centre
University of Manchester

This is a welcomed and extraordinary work on two counts. First, it is as close as one can get to the front-lines of the HIV/AIDS epidemic in the United States. Second, the epidemic in the U.S. is today as hidden and as denied as it is in China, Botswana and any place in the third world. Yet the investigators in these chapters found and recorded its dimensions, which makes this an extraordinary political and methodological achievement. Let me say more about why we in the international community especially welcome this work.

Since the beginning of the AIDS epidemic during the Reagan administration, we have watched the U.S. government, despite its extraordinary resources and wealth of talented public health expertise, serve as an example to the rest of the world of what not to do to prevent the spread of AIDS. We see what happens when a government responds to a dangerous communicable disease by criminal sanctions, withdrawal rather than expansion of vital community health services and refusal to take practical actions to reduce the harm that HIV and AIDS pose to the overall public health. The Bush administration policies leave us amazed that, contrary to the best scientific counsel in the world, moral persuasion is posed as an effective way to prevent the spread of a world pandemic. We have great respect for our colleagues in the U.S. scientific and public health communities for their quiet struggle against attempts to turn the clock and a great nation back to the middle ages in its public health practices. In this political climate, it is all the more extraordinary that the studies in this book were done and are now available to us. What you will read in city after city and in the U.S. Virgin Islands are dispassionate descriptions of the people and communities that constitute the front-lines of the HIV/AIDS epidemic in the United States. You will also learn that the lines are moving and that new high risk groups are emerging.

Predictably, the HIV/AIDS epidemic in the U.S. has been slowed and managed by more affluent Americans, but due to government inaction, it has been allowed to more rapidly advance among the poor and stigmatized. One outcome of such neglect, that we know to avoid in Europe based upon the U.S. example, is to have a dangerous disease driven into underground and hidden sub-populations such as injection drug users, sex traders, the criminalized unemployed, the homeless and youth who are without homes and living on the streets. None of these people are completely isolated from the general population and, if a dangerous communicable disease is allowed to spread among them, it is only a matter of time before it will re-emerge stronger and more dangerous in the larger public. Several chapters in this book have already described the bridges by which the epidemic is re-exposing an unsuspecting public to HIV. Once a disease is driven underground it is doubly hard to prevent and to monitor and poses great harm to the general public.

Underground sub-populations in the U.S., sometimes called the "underclass," are growing in size and complexity right in the midst of the most affluent nation on earth. Their evolving size and complexity are also measures of the extent to which they are hidden from public view and attention, more often, in plain sight. Standard random survey and interview techniques are not effective since these sub-populations cannot be enumerated. Here, some other way to glimpse the scope and character of the epidemic is needed. The chapters in this book are extraordinary not only because the political times do not favor action on the investigators' modest recommendations, they are extraordinary because they were able to systematically get the information presented here. They used the Rapid Assessment methodology which has been around for some time and used very effectively in public health studies of African and Asian impoverished communities. These American investigators in this book have adopted this methodology and now present us with the first American studies using Rapid Assessment.

It is ironic that a research technique had to be imported from the third world to study communities in the United States. But in terms of their social organization and day-to-day struggle to materially and emotionally survive, the underclass in the United States looks more and more like impoverished communities in the third world. It is another irony that there is concern in the United States for diseases developing in impoverished Asian and African communities that have potential to be carried via air travel with dangerous consequences to Los Angeles, New York or Chicago. Yet, in all of these cities and increasingly in rural communities as well, HIV continues with virtually no attention and effective prevention. The studies within are pioneering because they are the first systematic use of Rapid Assessment in the United States that is national in scope and because they will serve as models of subsequent studies of hidden subpopulations and communities in the United States. In order to understand all of the other social and public health issues affecting hidden people and communities, Rapid Assessment is a cost efficient and timely method for generating rich description and insight about human social life with difficult-to-reach people and places.

I found these studies to be very informative and sobering and hope that public health communities in the United States will be able to one day effectively end both the poverty that fans communicable diseases and the HIV/AIDS epidemic as well. Even if one day a vaccine and medical antidote are developed, it will be necessary to have the political will and resources to reach those at the far margins of American society. The chapters in this book tell us who they are and where they are.

Chapter 1

Exploring the Boundaries of the AIDS Epidemic in the U.S.

Ernest Quimby
Merrill Singer
Benjamin P. Bowser

What Should You Expect?

Our book provides a glimpse, a fleeting snapshot at best, of how socially constructed realities can be studied to minimize social catastrophe. Our focus is on AIDS, which is at once both a natural and manmade catastrophe on a global scale. At the risk of resorting to a cliché, AIDS is a chronic disease for some, but a pronouncement of death for others. Each chapter of *When Communities Assessing Their AIDS Epidemics* is both a stand-alone assessment, and a segment of the larger story of community response to AIDS in the U.S. This book includes studies that cover a range of communities from the supposedly idyllic U.S. Virgin Islands, to very troubled urban metropolises, to seemingly laid-back neighborhoods. The tone is not meant to be value-free or objective—especially when such alleged neutrality amounts to a subjective stance of condoning and accepting the status quo. It is, however, objective in the larger sense of using sound, qualitative methods to understand what is going on at ground-level in the AIDS epidemic.

As authors we are clearly partisans. We intend to stimulate thought and action to help wage a war that annually gets frontline coverage on World AIDS Day, but then recedes into selective amnesia for far too many of us.

However, our book is not an ideological pamphlet. It is the outgrowth of years of careful, critical, even skeptical scientific investigation based on a sound tradition of ethnography. We systematically illustrate, and explain where and how the epidemic is securing its most severe casualties, and generating collateral damage. Then we offer thoughtful and evidence-based recommendations.

Rather than provide the typical summaries of each chapter in this introduction, it may be more important to note the themes we are covering, and their significance. What you will read both reflects and results from a discomforting historical paradox and cliché—the more things change, the more they seem to remain the same. Yet the act of changing creates a new set of circumstances. As HIV/AIDS continues to exert its staggering toll, seemingly detached people and organizations have apparently become blasé, and almost stoical in their acceptance of this specter in our midst. AIDS has slipped into acceptance as one more chronic disease—like asthma, diabetes, and cancer—another unavoidable cost of modern life. What then are the social causes of AIDS (or asthma, diabetes, and cancer for that matter)? Are these not diseases we actually can do something about, yet seem not to, at least not in ways that equally benefit all those in harm's way?

Instead we are still haunted, and stalked. Back in the nineteen eighties, seemingly a generation or so ago when the virus was detected, some individuals were self-comforted by their socially constructed realities and cocoons. For them, AIDS was a disease that 'those people' get.

The realization emerged then, and only after protracted struggles by its victims and their allies. This thing, this awful and dreadful horror, was relentless, merciless, remorseless, and resourceful. Anyone could be afflicted; it could even get to "me." Nevertheless, the definitions and perceptions of the media, government, religious, medical, and social sectors that regarded HIV/AIDS as ruthless is still focused on the highest risk groups—white gays, needle-using drug addicts and prostitutes. For a while, even Haitians were thrown into the risk basket of 'Social Others.' For the rest of us, HIV/AIDS was a dread to be reckoned with vicariously, perhaps when a deviant relative or friend was diagnosed. Otherwise, we were safe and life could go on as before.

Social and personal myths were devised, furthering the wedge between acknowledgment and responsibility, acceptance and action, words and deeds, death and life. As the disease ripped asunder the social fabric of African American communities, exacting untold pain and suffering, the Congressional Black Caucus appealed to the U.S. Health and Human Services Administration to declare HIV/AIDS a national emergency in large black metropolitan areas. For a moment they were successful. A number of cities declared emergencies and did update studies of their epidemic, but were unable to implement recommendations or do follow-up studies without continued federal funding. This national failure symbolizes our failure to fully grasp the impact of the epidemic on low income communities and people of color. Certain questions were unavoidably raised: What must be done? And by whom? How, when, and where can we start?

This book summarizes the initial studies that came out of the 1998 HIV/AIDS state of emergency and provides answers to the above questions. It presents descriptions of an effective qualitative methodology, shares extensive findings and offers numerous practical and necessary recommendations to stem the HIV onslaught. When affected communities are equipped and trained to assess the paths, targets and consequences of HIV/AIDS in their midst, then a realm of life-saving public policies can be implemented to alter the progression of this disease.

To address the HIV/AIDS health crisis in African America, a national Rapid Assessment, Response and Evaluation (RARE) initiative was launched in 1999 in response to the effort of the Congressional Black Caucus. It was designed to link people on the ground with access to the highest risk groups with professional researchers. The following chapters contain perspectives, experiences, data, findings, conclusions, and recommendations resulting from this endeavor.

What Were Our Research Questions?

RARE teams around the country had several measurable objectives: to collaboratively, efficiently, and expeditiously detect the disease's main local trajectory, and to answer core behavioral and contextual questions concerning local factors that were contributing to the continued spread of HIV infection. This involved identifying neighborhood risk hot spots and describing risky behaviors and their participants. A related, deeper, emergent level of inquiry centered on the disease's progression, and the effects of the shattered political economies of local communities to spread the disease further. Accordingly, the analysis focused on structural associations between sites, observed activities, and broader institutional issues described in our conclusion.

The RARE methodology is qualitative; it is intent upon discovering insights about the epidemic, and its course rather than quantitatively measuring what we already know. We also made attempts to make connections, build real and affirming relationships between researchers and people in the affected neighborhoods. The traditional power paradigm, the dynamic of research subjects, and (master) researchers were shifted to one of active participation in planning, data collection, analysis, evaluation, and policy changes by those most affected by AIDS in both its biological and social dimensions. Despite the long tradition of ethnography, RARE was viewed by some as an insurrectionist approach. Not only was it a means of collecting data, but also of incorporating procedures rooted in the philosophy that local peoples can and should define their problems, and their relations.

Our book articulates some of the unheard voices of the AIDS epidemic both from within and outside the AIDS establishment. Despite, or perhaps because of levels of fear and confusion, community and national organizers formed alliances with researchers and policy makers who recognized the urgent need for new ways of obtaining, and using health data. Information has traditionally been top down, i.e., based on the perspectives and methodologies of scientists, policy makers and government officials who tend to be removed from the communities most ravished by HIV/AIDS. The results have been obvious and tragic. Missed opportunities for prevention and treatment have led to a worsening situation.

One documented theme that emerges from this experience is the crucial need to appreciate the political economics of HIV/AIDS transmission. Meaningful epidemiology encompasses, even demands, the integration of bio-medical and sociological factors. This fact has not been recognized sufficiently. The devastating consequences of the political and economic contexts in which HIV/AIDS exists, (e.g., historical processes of globalization, economic transformations and community destabilization), have led to structural insufficiencies in the capacities of local municipalities to protect themselves. Other major challenges in this battle include marginalizing people politically, the cultural contexts of the epidemic, and the lack of reliable scientific data, especially the availability of such data in a workable form that communities can use to address their AIDS crisis. Racism, homophobia, stigma, and rejection of drug users deemed to be illicit, have all conspired against working class, and poor neighborhoods. Distrust by community residents, competing personal and social problems, ignored or ignorant leadership, moral condemnation, denial, and lack of sustained mobilization have all contributed to a lack of proactive prevention of HIV/AIDS.

When Communities Assessing Their AIDS Epidemics is a pioneering effort that offers three important examples. We show how applied qualitative research can be useful at the community level, how a qualitative research methodology can be empowering, and how a qualitative methodology can also be used as an instrument of social policy. These points will become evident as you read each chapter, revealing both the shared features and unique ways the RARE method was adapted to fit the unique conditions of each social setting.

What Were Our Methods and Data Sources?

We used geo-mapping, field observations, focus groups, in-depth individual interviews, and street intercepts. These methods are described, and critically analyzed as they were applied in each city and their communities. Care is taken not to over-generalize. Since RARE's beginning, specially trained Crisis Response Teams (CRTs) of community residents have conducted literally thousands of hours of investigation. Among the people observed and/or interviewed were business proprietors, sex workers, youth, drug dealers, drug users, persons living with AIDS, ex-offenders, service providers, persons with a mental disorder, and homeless individuals. Participants, both adult and juvenile, were selected to ensure diversity in racial, national, age, cultural, and gender orientation. Participants included self-identified heterosexuals, gays, lesbians, males who have sex with males, bi-sexuals, and transgender persons.

What Are RARE's Pitfalls?

Although a considerable improvement over other approaches, the RARE model is not heralded here as a panacea for all existing conceptual and methodological problems confronting community AIDS research. As the following chapters will attest, sometimes we did encounter shortcomings. Several of those can be summarized as follows:

- Aspects of initial team training lacked depth, and were too brief;
- Local health departments were not uniformly and clearly committed to the project;
- At times, team training was minimized because of their confused roles within the health department;
- Team training did not consistently emphasize data analysis;
- The roles, objectives, relationships, and tasks among federal health officials, local health officials, and field teams were not always specified and clarified;
- Advisory boards did not exist or operate at all sites;
- At times, local health department staff were not available for an initial meeting with the lead researchers and team, although the project was expected to be completed within eight to ten weeks;
- Fieldwork was sometimes interrupted for various reasons, including changes in health staff, financial issues, unresolved institutional review board requirements, and delays in hiring or paying team members;
- CRT members needed to appreciate and accept the differences between research and service. They were advised to avoid promising services after the research ended. Yet the tension between conducting data collection, and their desire to serve led some team members to make promises to participants that should not have been made. Some teams resolved some of their discomfort by passing out condoms and literature while they were in the field, but they were instructed to refrain from making promises of service delivery following the research;
- A lack of central health department focus, structure, direction, and leadership created significant challenges for fieldwork. This was especially illustrated by some team members' frustration, and low morale because of chronically late and incomplete paychecks, and unresolved fiscal issues between the local health department, community vendor, logistical contractor, and the federal RARE office;
- Technical assistance from the logistical contractor was sometimes delayed;
- Ethnographic training (re: philosophy, purpose, rationale, methods, process, analysis, and assessment) was needed for local health officials, and advisory committee members. A special training session was some-

times needed for them to fully understand the nature, and scope of the work to be undertaken, but it was not provided;

- Training for the field team about the local health department's related initiatives, policies, and programs was not generally provided. Prior to the fieldwork, ethnographers did not consistently receive orientation and background information pertaining to the status of the local health department's HIV/AIDS programs, policies, and initiatives in the designated sites. This would have allowed the ethnographers to give more direct, and insightful assistance to the field team. Knowledge of the research context is essential.

How Did We Apply RARE Modules?

Despite these shortcomings, RARE had much potential and notable success. The following chapters document clearly its strengths as a data collection, and analysis procedure, and its methodology for developing evidence-based policy recommendations. The transition process from the initial RARE field team training to the actual fieldwork module was facilitated greatly by weekly meetings. At each site the local field teams met regularly, sometimes with representatives from the local health department, to iron out their problems, and define awaiting tasks. As team members began a twenty-four hour cycle of observations of the neighborhoods, each meeting began with a review of observations and was followed by additional instruction. Training included both planned assignments and discussions of topics raised during weekly meetings.

Modules were applied in the following order: direct observation, geo-mapping, street intercepts, focus groups, and in-depth interviews. The direct observations and geo-mapping provided insight into what was taking place in the community, where it was taking place, and who was participating in the activities/behaviors of concern. Street intercepts provided information on why things were occurring. Focus groups and in-depth interviews allowed for a deeper probing to understand the social contexts of what we observed.

Different city sites regarded some modules more effective than others. For some teams, the most potent module was direct observation. For others, focus groups and in-depth interviews generated the most meaningful information in the quickest time.

How Did We Organize Our Data?

Generally, each site held a debriefing session at each meeting. Each team leader reported the team's activities for the week, the patterns of observed behavior, new observations, and what the team expected to do in the next week. Members commented on the weekly report, and noted any similarities, and differences in team members' work. When there was confirmation of a consistently reported behavior or activity by varied methods of data collection, i.e., triangulation, the information would constitute a finding. Data were initially categorized according to the following:

- Types of risky behaviors and activities;
- The location of hot spots for risky behaviors and activities;
- Peak times for risky behaviors and activities;
- Types of outreach programs observed on the streets, if any;
- Who participates in the risky behaviors and activities;
- Reasons for participating in the behaviors and activities;
- Types of preventive materials and programs available in communities;
- Barriers that prevent access to treatment and prevention;
- Community members' knowledge and perceptions of HIV/AIDS causes, treatments, and prevention measures.

The subsequent arrangement of data into emergent themes led to conclusions about the debilitating effects of the political economies of most affected neighborhoods. The lessons learned resulted both from the process, and resulting data about issues that were insufficiently clear at the onset of the RARE project. These data-driven conceptual categories are described in each chapter, and in the Conclusion. They include discovery of new HIV risk sites; where AIDS-related knowledge is lacking; where pressing interventions are needed; what local decision-makers were lacking; and identification of barriers to change, and reinvigoration of HIV/AIDS prevention efforts.

In all of the local site studies, recommendations evolved from a process that began with findings from direct observations, and geo-mapping (which identified the where, when, and what), and was continued with in-depth interviews, and street intercepts that lent deeper insight into who and why. Based upon team members' observations, and findings, recommendations were developed, reviewed, and finalized. The goal was to develop achievable recommendations that did not require longer-term and sweeping social changes, but rather those that could be accomplished by local communities with existing resources.

Implementation has been mixed. At the negative extreme, to date one local health department, despite inquiries, has not acknowledged a final field research report, and no advisory board or community-working group exists for review and feedback. The internal politics of the local health department seem to prohibit serious consideration of the findings and recommendations. At the positive end of the spectrum, official municipal reaction has been embracing and appreciative. Recommendations have been acted upon and incorporated into local public health policies. There has been a careful, considerate, and straightforward adoption of some recommendations.

Why Read This Book?

This book should be read judiciously, studied, and shared for many reasons. Four reasons may be cited at this point. First, our book illustrates why a grasp of political economy and an appreciation for historical aspects of community destabilization are essential to understanding the contexts in which HIV/AIDS thrives. When people and neighborhoods are marginalized, socially quarantined, and abandoned, they become ever more vulnerable to a disease whose containment requires accurate information, political commitment, considerable resources, and fundamental changes in social structures, social relations, attitudes, and behaviors. One of the central lessons of RARE is that HIV/AIDS is about power and structured social inequality. Failure to grasp this point has placed many people at avoidable risk, and has needlessly caused loss of life.

Second, the HIV and AIDS rates of African Americans and Latinos remain high, particularly for people, behaviors, and neighborhoods identified during our research. *When Communities Assessing Their AIDS Epidemic* includes information on city, and site-specific social contexts, findings, lessons learned, and recommendations. It offers a unique opportunity for academicians, policymakers, researchers, and frontline workers to learn from and build upon our strategies. Replication of our efforts can contribute to HIV/AIDS reduction, and prevention in other communities.

Third, our project's strengths include highly informed and interdisciplinary teams, access to HIV-vulnerable and politically disenfranchised hot spots, identification of significant findings, and presentation of well-grounded recommendations. The challenges, the RARE project shows, are accessing resources, balancing research and service, and negotiating with health officials to engage in effective follow-up based upon doable recommendations.

Fourth, our book is a testimony from the margins of American society. It attempts to articulate aspects of our socially, and structurally constructed realities which perpetuate the AIDS epidemic. We are in a decisive struggle, not just to contain a particular disease, but to alter the way we live. Because RARE was based on qualitative methods, it allows the reader to move beyond the usual mountain of AIDS statistics to confront, and transcend the cultural shields that hide the faces of real human beings grappling daily with pressing personal and social issues. In the end, their faces, and ours are the same in this time of AIDS.

Chapter 2

Rapid Assessment: A Method for Community-Based Research

Robert T. Trotter, II
Merrill Singer

Introduction

The RARE method was used to conduct the research presented in this book and is what makes this work unique in its depth and richness. For those who are unfamiliar with RARE, this chapter describes the method in detail. RARE is part of a series of innovations in research methods that is relatively new to the United States. Rapid assessment has become a standard data collection and policy development tool for the World Health Organization (WHO) (Rhodes et al. 1999, Fitch and Stimpson 2003), the U.S. Department of Health and Human Services (DHHS) (Needle et al. 2003, Trotter and Needle 1999, Singer 2000), as well as international, regional and local governments. Rapid assessment is being promoted as a fast, easy, community-controlled research design that will solve time-sensitive problems for HIV and AIDS programs in both developing countries and in hard-to-reach populations in the developed world (Singer 1999, Trotter and Needle 1999).

Rapid assessment is also being promoted by the Centers for Disease Control and Prevention (CDC) and the U.S. National Institutes of Health (NIH) as being cheaper and less time-intensive than standard survey techniques, and some epidemiological approaches to HIV-related problems (Needle et al. 2000). These promotions for rapid assessment can be seen either as scientifically based or hyperbole, depending on the soundness of the design, adequacy of the training for personnel, rigor of the quality control, and degree of sophistication of the analytical capacity that are fielded at the local level where the rapid assessment is being conducted.

Brief History

Rapid ethnographic assessment originally evolved from the research designs of traditional ethnographic research (Bernard 1998, Scrimshaw 1987). This innovation was created to take advantage of advancements in mid-range ethnographic theory (Trotter 1997), systematic sampling, and a growing enthusiasm for the involvement of local communities in public health research, planning, intervention and action. "Rapid assessment" was first described in the mid-1980s (Scrimshaw et al. 1987, 1991, Scrimshaw and Gleason 1992, Bentley et al. 1988).

There are other parallel rapid assessment and evaluation procedures that developed simultaneously, such as rural rapid appraisal and participatory action research (Dale et al. 1996, Heaver 1991, Lee and Price 1995, Malilay 1997, Whyte 1995). All of these approaches attempt to shorten the time from data collection to policy development without losing the rigor and defensibility of less rapid scientific processes. From inception, rapid assessment has coupled ethnographic theory with extensive local cultural knowledge and involvement (Scrimshaw and Hurtado 1987, Bentley et al. 1988, Scrimshaw and Gleason 1992).

A brief survey of recent rapid assessment projects shows that a very wide variety of issues and complex community conditions has been addressed with rapid assessment research. These include infectious diseases from malaria to diarrheal disease (Alemedon 1997, Askew et al. 1993, Ayepong 1995) disaster intervention (Malilay et al. 1997), disabilities research (Trotter et al. 2001), assessment of district health program needs (Materia et al. 1995), pregnant women and sexually transmitted disease in Thailand (Kilmarx et al. 1996), and drug use (Perry et al. 1999). This flexibility is one of the strengths and one of the selling points of rapid assessment in community settings. The research agenda can be very much locally structured and controlled.

RARE's Goals

The goal of the rapid assessment process is to provide the necessary information for the local community to make informed decisions about the local health and social problems, the kinds of interventions that are required, the resources that are needed, and the types of programs that are acceptable to the community. Participants understand from the project's inception that any local response will be influenced by social, cultural, political, religious, ethical and economic factors. Interventions will have to be made locally acceptable and feasible. This suggests that rapid assessments should only be undertaken at times and in places where there is already a commitment to do something (i.e., to make identified programmatic, policy, or procedural changes that will help to lower risk or expand care). However, rapid assessments can also be used to alert leaders and local organizations to new problems or to critical changes in existing problems where actions and new responses are needed.

Basic Descriptions of the Core Methods

Rapid assessment is a combination of several qualitative research techniques aimed at deriving new information and insights about hard-to-reach or access groups. The technique is flexible enough to integrate quantitative research approaches as well. Information is acquired in such a way that it can be conveniently used by government and local social service and health agencies to address quickly and effectively any social and health problems. The basic methods suite for rapid assessment is very well described, and has evolved out of basic (Bernard 1998) and applied (Trotter and Schenshul 1998; WHO 1998a, 1998b; Stimpson et al. 1999; Scrimshaw 1991; Trotter and Needle 1999) qualitative research models. The specific model for the U.S. DHHS design for rapid assessment is called RARE (Rapid Assessment, Response, and Evaluation) and is presented in this chapter.

There are five basic qualitative methods combined in the RARE method. They are:

1. Individual Qualitative Interviews

Who is Interviewed

Individual qualitative interviews are called key informant interviews in the ethnographic methods literature. Key informants are people from the target group who have special awareness of a topic that interests the researcher. Key informants are "cultural experts" who are not only knowledgeable, but are willing and able to share the information of interest with the researcher. Most frequently, they are highly respected experts, and are able to describe and discuss key issues about their culture. They can provide special insights into both the processes and the rationale for what people do, why they do it, how they do it, where, when, and with whom they do it. Key informants serve as cultural consultants to the data collection process, helping to insure access to target group members, sites, and information. Key informants are also individuals who show up on a minimum of four expert lists because of their knowledge, achievements, and regard in their community.

How It Is Done

Key informant interviews are open-ended, conversationally styled research interviews that explore knowledge, beliefs, values, experiences, and understanding in depth. These interviews are normally structured by a series of broad questions from a general question guide. The experienced interviewer encourages the discussion to be controlled by the cultural expert rather than the interviewer. This allows the interview to generate new information and new knowledge that the interviewer may not know beforehand which is relevant and important to the project. This discovery process is a major advantage of key informant interviews over surveys that can focus on only known information. For example, when the following questions about people, place and time with regard to HIV risk behaviors are answered by the data, the key informant interviews have been successfully completed.

HIV Risk

- Who are the vulnerable populations?
- What are the different patterns of risk and protective behaviors, access and use of services that influence transmission of HIV, progression to AIDS, and morbidity and mortality associated with behaviors and HIV/AIDS?
- Which subgroups are at greatest/lowest risk of acquiring HIV, progressing to AIDS, experiencing morbidity and mortality associated with behaviors?
- What is the extent of HIV risk, HIV infection and AIDS in subgroups at risk (gender and by exposure group) in the community?
- What are the extent, availability and accessibility for subgroups, relative to their risk for HIV, progression to HIV/AIDS and morbidity/mortality?

Context of HIV Risk

- What are the local norms, values, beliefs that influence HIV risk and protective behaviors, access, and use of services?
- What and where are the locations/settings in which behaviors occur that influence patterns that influence risk and protective behaviors?
- How do the settings (physical environment and socio-cultural context) influence the patterns of risk and protective behaviors?
- What is the extent and availability of existing interventions, treatment and care?
- What are the factors that increase/decrease likelihood of changing risk behaviors, and/or sustaining protective behaviors?

Type of Interventions

- What are the extent, availability and accessibility of existing prevention interventions, and treatment and care services?

- Who is being served and how are they being reached?
- What is the socio-cultural appropriateness of the interventions and services?
- What are the advantages and disadvantages of the existing interventions and services?
- What is working and needs to be continued, expanded, and adapted for different groups?
- What is not working and has to be discontinued?
- What intervention strategies have not been implemented?

2. Focus Groups

Focus groups are qualitative, in-depth, group interviews that explore key cultural information in an interactive format. They are similar to key informant interviews except they are designed to capture the interactions between people, and differences in opinion. This is in addition to the cultural consensus that is present in the group. Focus groups are characterized by the use of a natural language format (conversational style questions) that allows the controlled exploration of a topic. The strengths of focus groups are that they encourage open discussion and they explore differences of opinion that are not apparent in most one-on-one interviews. Focus groups generally produce a greater breadth of coverage when compared to key informant interviews.

Focus groups fall into a small number of types. One type, called the Exploratory Model, is excellent for exploring topics for which there is little information available. This type allows researchers to examine unknown cultural domains in some depth with a group of cultural experts. In exploratory focus groups, the facilitator focuses on trying to get participants to freely discuss topics about which little is known, while noting items for more intensive probing and exploration, either later in the focus group or in follow-up interviews and observations.

Another type of focus group, called the KAB Model (knowledge, attitudes and beliefs), emphasizes the exploration and clarification of community attitudes about issues, in addition to beliefs and knowledge. Here, the facilitator tries to keep the group "on track" in its discussion, rather than mixing together attitudes, beliefs, and behaviors. The facilitator's goal is to get full and detailed accounts in all three of the cultural elements of concern.

Finally, there is the focus group type called the Consumer Model that is used especially for evaluating a product or an idea, for developing interview questions for a survey, and for validating findings from other research processes. One use of the Consumer Model is to test community response to a planned community intervention program. Hence, the participants could be presented with an intervention approach suggested by rapid assessment and then asked to share their attitudes toward this approach, including their opinions about its appropriateness for the target group(s).

All three of these types of focus groups help to identify intra-cultural variation in people's knowledge and experience. Also, each type of focus group allows researchers to explore qualitative content richly, observe the interactions between people while they are discussing topics of interest, and describe how people discuss a particular topic. They also help to assure the researcher that key topics or issues are not ignored.

There are both advantages and disadvantages to using focus groups in rapid assessment. Some savings in cost and time is one of the advantages. One focus group takes about the same time as two good key informant interviews, and allows a topic to be explored with eight to ten different people in that timeframe. Also, it provides information on issues, not just a single viewpoint. Focus groups have two primary disadvantages. First, they reduce an individual's opportunity to go into depth on a topic. Everyone has to have time to speak, so no one can provide all of the information they have. Second, people do not always state what they really believe when doing so in public. Sometimes they say only what they think is acceptable to the group, whereas in a one-on-one interview, they feel greater freedom to express their own opinion, even if it is not one that is widely shared. However, by using both key informant interviews and focus groups together, the advantages of each can be strengthened, and the disadvantages of both can be minimized.

3. Observations

The RARE method suite provides methodological information and training on direct observation techniques to complement the interview methods described above. Observation is naturalistic, in that it is done, commonly, in the normal day-to-day settings and with the target group. As noted by the World Health Organization (WHO 1998, 1999), observation "allows the researcher to gain first-hand experience of human behavior, meanings, relationships, and contexts. The observer learns by being present, by seeing what people do, and by listening to what they say." Observation can also complement other research methods.

In RARE, observation was used initially to:

- Describe locations for research (e.g., risk pockets), geo-map key areas, facilitate field team access to local risk sites and identify key informants;
- Identify and provide naturalistic and detailed accounts of risk behaviors and risk contexts.

Later in the data-collection process, observation was more commonly used to:

- Validate and cross-check findings from other methods (i.e., triangulation);

- Further explore specific topics, groups, or behaviors of concern;
- Assess the representativeness of the emerging findings achieved through repeating observations with different groups in different areas;
- Spot potential problems and possible solutions for action plan recommendations.

These observations were then written up or transferred to maps and were used as part of the data triangulation process to complete the RARE project findings and recommendations. Observations were particularly important in selecting risk sites for greater concentration on key issues, using the other methods. They also contributed to the construction of questions of local relevance based on actual, on-the-ground behaviors and settings.

4. Mapping

The use of 'mapping' techniques was valuable in RARE for exploring the "territory" of risk and the physical context in which that risk exists. Mapping also assisted in generating theories and ideas for further research, and in validating existing findings. At the start of a rapid assessment, the field teams were sometimes unsure of what they should be observing, and where these observations should take place. By conducting a mapping exercise in the area in which the rapid assessment was to take place, teams were given both a focus point to discuss and a location for their observations. Written descriptions of potential HIV risk locations are useful, but maps can provide visual representations of complex information. Mapping can also be used to monitor where interviews have taken place or can help focus group participants to highlight areas that would benefit from a prevention project. Observational methods can be used to supplement maps by identifying where the key locations and individuals are in an area. Mapping was utilized in RARE projects to achieve the following goals:

- *Collect data*—maps that illustrate aspects of the physical and social environment in which HIV risk occurs, and where prevention and intervention are offered.
- *Present data*—maps that distill information into clear graphical overviews.
- *Understand data*—maps that also help to highlight trends or relationships that were not obvious or fully understood (time-based maps) at the beginning of the study.
- *Plan action*—maps that help to plan intervention activities and track them over time.

The RARE training manuals emphasize the following types of maps that are useful to RARE projects:

- Locations where people gather and risks take place—bars, drug treatment clinics, shooting galleries, drug dealing locations, places where syringes or condoms are sold on the street, prostitution stroll areas, parks, and secluded places.
- Locations of other indicators—this could include locations where discarded syringes and condoms are found.
- Boundaries affecting assessment—boundary areas that separate two different social groups (e.g., ethnic neighborhoods) may be of special importance as "mixing" areas where different populations (and their drug-use patterns) interact.
- Main zones of activity of community-based organizations (CBOs)—these are the catchment areas or usual focus areas for CBO service agencies.

5. Surveys

The option for rapid assessment surveys was built into the basic RARE methodology tool kit to allow sites to explore and answer questions that were raised, but not completely answered by the qualitative methods. These surveys, sometimes called street surveys, were designed to take no more than five minutes, to be anonymous, and to consist of no more than ten questions. Questions can be quantitative in nature, and while other questions can be open-ended, qualitative questions. The basic idea is to be able to go to a targeted site and randomly sample individuals at that location to ask them specific questions about a location and what happens there. This type of survey was necessary in only a small portion of the RARE projects, because, in the end, the other data collection tools provided more than sufficient information to design locally sensitive programs, policies, and interventions.

The RARE Methodological Suite

Goal Assumptions

The RARE model has been constructed to meet a series of goals. First, it assumes that RARE projects will complement existing data sets, procedures and epidemiological knowledge rather than be a "stand alone" effort. The following goals characterize well-constructed RARE projects.

1. Speed: A well-targeted RARE project can be accomplished in approximately twelve weeks from implementation to release of action plans. In

practice, local contexts present a range of shared and unique challenges that may cause a RARE project to take longer to complete.

2. Non-duplicative: RARE complements ongoing processes, more than it replaces them. It allows a more tightly targeted focus for information collection when compared with broad area statistical or planning data collection. In domains where there is no data or only very limited data collection, RARE offers policy-relevant data.
3. Triangulation: The use of multiple methods and multiple data sources increases the validity and defensibility of the results. This aspect of the RARE process responds to concerns about the use of qualitative data sources for policy decisions; RARE is predicated on the assumption that validity is enhanced when several different methods produce similar results.
4. Focus on contexts and situations: RARE makes it possible to discover solutions that fit local contexts. This means being culturally specific and able to accommodate local values and conditions based on work carried out by people from the local setting.
5. Local Involvement and Community Consultation: RARE is designed to be conducted and owned at a local level, to involve a broad network of local participants in the decision-making and oversight process, and to involve staff from existing community organizations and institutions.
6. Pragmatic: RARE is designed to be closely targeted, and not to do everything for everyone. The approach produces practical and pragmatic recommendations based upon local conditions and what needs to be done to change those conditions.
7. Based on Local Cultural Knowledge: The RARE approach enfranchises cultural experts who have both local perspective and the methodological expertise to provide a valid and reliable evaluation of data collected through rapid assessment techniques. Local cultural knowledge extends beyond the community to include specific life knowledge and experience in various local neighborhoods, with locally available ethnic groups and other social groupings (e.g., street gangs, illicit drug users, people with HIV, etc.).

Critical Issues

The most critical methodological issue to be addressed in the RARE suite is the extent to which findings have more than a superficial validity. To outline RARE's potential as well as its limits, it is necessary to discuss sampling and triangulation.

Sampling

One of the most commonly asked questions about a rapid assessment project is, "How many people have to be interviewed and observed to provide good data?" There is no straightforward answer to this question. RARE projects use well-established, qualitative sampling designs, or a combination of qualitative and quantitative samples. Several texts have focused on qualitative sampling (Johnson 1990, Kuzel 1992; Luborsky and Rubinstein 1995). Other works describe how to combine qualitative and quantitative sampling (cf. Miller and Payne 1993; Johnson 1990). The framework for the RARE sampling approach provides a complimentary design that allows for both qualitative and quantitative samples to be judiciously and simultaneously collected as part of the assessment process.

It is important to note that the construction of qualitative samples is guided by a different set of rules than those governing the development of quantitative samples. Quantitative samples are meant to be estimation samples, while the majority of qualitative samples are designed to be cultural saturation samples. Estimation samples allow the researcher to extrapolate larger population characteristics from much smaller sets. On the other hand, cultural saturation samples allow the researcher to describe more thoroughly the cultural consensus (beliefs that are widely shared), and the variability of beliefs within a population.

In qualitative research, the ideal procedure for assuring adequate sample size is to interview to redundancy (i.e., until no new or unexplained elements or conditions of the cultural domain have been exposed in new interviews). However, practical applications of rapid assessment have demonstrated that "pragmatic redundancy," that is, sufficient information to provide confidence in the data, can be achieved long before total redundancy occurs. This is possible because most qualitative interviews with local cultural experts often contain the core cultural beliefs, values and contextual information that are available in the overall population. This approach produces a strong description of cultural consensus and the majority of variation in views and sentiments within a high risk group.

It is not effective or efficient to talk to people who do not know enough about their situation to provide good advice on policy or program changes. Frequently, the gold standard in quantitative research, a random sample, is an inefficient way of producing comprehensive information about a cultural domain. Most randomly selected individuals have limited knowledge of the subject. They all too often are asked to describe what they do not know, rather than what they actually do know. In contrast with the limits of quantitative sampling, there are two qualitative sampling frames that are more successful (Van Meter 1990, Sudman and Kalton 1986; Sudman et al. 1986; Johnson 1990):

1. Nominated samples are derived from asking those who know a culture and its inhabitants to nominate people to be interviewed who have in-depth knowledge and experience of that population. For example, the best "cultural experts" to nominate in a place where there is AIDS risk among men who have sex with men are the long-time popular leaders in the local gay community.

2. Targeted sampling is used where nominated frameworks are not feasible or where a broader geographical sample is needed. They also are used to

find the people who can designate individuals for a nominated sampling frame. Targeted samples are constructed by determining the categories of individuals who are likely to have the most knowledge and experience about a cultural domain and who represent the most likely variation in experience with that cultural area. These samples are also assembled by selecting people within specified physical locations such as a housing complex, block, or some HIV risk venue. In many cases, targeted sampling is used to find individuals who are representatives of hidden or very rare populations (Singer 1999; Braunstein 1993; Griffiths 1993; Sudman et al. 1988).

The RARE project combines these sampling approaches to construct samples that are appropriate to the core methods. In our project, nominated samples were used to collect information from a combination of community leaders, service providers, and people vulnerable to HIV infection. Targeted and geo-targeted frameworks were used to collect samples for the direct observational methods, brief cultural domain interviews and the rapid assessment surveys for RARE. These approaches were judged to have the highest probability of providing the most defensible and comprehensive data in a minimum amount of time.

Table 2.1

Table 2.1: Examples of Matching Methods and Sample Sizes for RARE Projects

Methods	Sample Frame	N
Key Informant Interviews	Nominated Cultural Expert Sample	15 per cultural domain,[1] per population segment[2]
Focus Groups	Nominated Cultural Expert Sample	3 groups, 8–10 people each, per cultural domain, per key population segment
Rapid Assessment Survey (Street Intercept)	Random selection within targeted community context	30 per key issue area, per key population segment
Direct Observation	Targeted Rapid Environmental Assessment Sampling to observe and identify all key sites and intervention-related behaviors	minimum – observation in 10 locations with 10 key informants

Triangulation

As noted previously, triangulation is a condition that contributes to reliability in mixed methods designs (Nickel et al. 1995; Bernard 1998). The configuration of methods used in RARE is designed to be a set of complimentary techniques selected to address a specific research problem. The mix should vary by the question that is being explored, the cultural context of the issue, and the types of applications that are expected from the project. Single methods, such as focus groups or key informant interviews, provide evidence of both consensual and conflicting views about a cultural domain. Adding other methods often helps explain the consensus and/or account for conflicts (e.g., when focus group members are in significant disagreement about something). For example, focus groups tend to produce "public" discourse and provide information about what people say they do or should be doing. When this is matched with direct field observations of the behavior discussed in the focus group, it is often possible to confirm some of the things that were said, and to discover variations between what people say they should do and their actual behavior. This helps researchers confirm complimentary data based upon methods of mixed data collection.

The following cultural data and methods matrix (table 2.2) identifies the ways in which the RARE core methods provide triangulation of information for a successful RARE project. The rows name a specific method, and the columns indicate whether or not there is a solid analytic strategy that will produce information from the data that can be used to sculpt an intervention or policy that is responsive both to community needs and to community sensitivities.

Table 2.2

Table 2.2: RARE Cultural Data and Methods Matrix

Methods	Beliefs Knowledge And Values	Risk Activities and	Physical Context and Structure	Symbols Language and Communication
Key Informant Interviews	yes	yes	yes	yes
Focus Groups	yes	yes	yes	yes
Geo-mapping		yes	yes	
Direct Obser-vation	yes	yes	yes	yes
Rapid Surveys and Short Street Inter-views	yes	yes	yes	yes
Natural Lan-guage and Communica-tion Explora-tion	yes	yes		yes

The Flaws of Rapid Assessment

Rapid assessment can be more vulnerable to surprises and serendipity than other methodologies without action and policy objectives. There can be conflicts among staff, insufficient time to build rapport before having to "get down to work," a mad scramble for quickly approaching deadlines, or an unanticipated lack of support from persons. All projects at some time face situations that work," a mad scramble for quickly approaching deadlines, or an unanticipated lack of support from persons. All projects at some time face situations that threaten the strength and usefulness of their findings and outcomes. The most common threats arise out of any one or combination of the following: 1) inadequately trained or inexperienced personnel; 2) poor or inadequate quality control; 3) logistics problems; 4) incorrect locations targeted for the use of rapid assessment designs, 5) poor analysis, and; 6) an inability to transform data and findings into achievable recommendations and action plans. All of these problems are enhanced by the short timeframe of this methodology, and the very limited budgets that are generally available. Despite these issues, those who use this methodology have generally found it to be effective and productive, even when there are limited resources. However, there are other more specific problems that can occur.

Incorrect Targeting

The initial design of a rapid assessment project is critical to its success. Rapid assessment works best when it has a specific target population, is defined narrowly in scope and is reasonably bound geographically. The political process through which the rapid assessment goals are defined often cause problems for a RARE project. Most failed projects were problematic at the start. These projects were dependent upon first addressing a local agenda; the research was secondary and is used to fulfill that agenda. Alternatively, the initial problem identification may have been too broad.

Communities with different interests are normally involved in identifying the primary focus for a RARE project. Since this is a political process, "stakeholders" such as health officials, community representatives, service providers, community-based organization staff, local political officials, and community leaders come together to decide what the target of a rapid assessment project should be. All these individuals rarely achieve a perfect consensus (Trotter and Needle 2001; WHO 1998). Nearly everyone in these groups has a clear and slightly different agenda and focus: whether it is youth, drug users, men who have sex with men, women, or any other group that has strong advocacy representation (or lack of representation) in the community. Therefore, care must be taken at this initial stage to focus the rapid assessment on appropriate needs, rather than simply on political expediency.

Inadequate Personnel and Quality Control

There is a simple rule for rapid assessment projects: they should not be conducted if there are no experienced ethnographers available to guide them. Many of the functions that are part of conducting a rapid assessment project can be filled by individuals who have received high-quality training before and during pal Investigator or P.I., for research projects). This person needs the broadest and deepest knowledge, skills and training in ethnographic methods of all the individuals on the project. This is the person responsible for translating the community's initial targeting and problem identification into sound rapid assessment questions, project design and field procedures. The P.I. also is responsible for overseeing the data collection process and providing quality control for the data that is collected. This means that the P.I. must supervise staff, assure adherence to project design, and check the completeness of the data assembled by the field team. Finally, the P.I. is the primary individual responsible for the appropriate analysis of the field data and the development of useful recommendations from that data. While some of the routine administrative functions of the project can be done by others, the quality of the P.I. is directly correlated with the quality of the data, the quality of the analysis, and the impact of the project's recommendations. This is no place for on-the-job training as an alternative to the a-priori possession of a high level of ethnographic research and analytic skills. Basic administrative skills are also needed.

Field personnel for rapid assessment projects are commonly recruited from existing agencies and community-based organizations based on their "street knowledge" of the community and/or target group. A positive reputation in the community also counts. Both qualities contribute significantly to project success. However, this diversity of "temporary" or short-term personnel creates a great need for logistical administration (scheduling, payroll, data storage and processing, etc.). Use of temporary staff increases the likelihood that some work will not get completed as planned or that staff will leave the project before it is completed. Also, temporary staff generally is less committed.

The choice of field personnel is the third crucial personnel feature of rapid assessment. Ethnographic methods work best when the individuals doing the data collection are familiar with and accepted by the community. Standard ethnographies are often conducted by individuals who begin as strangers to a community. But they have the commitment, communication skills, and time to become familiar, accepted, trusted and integrated into community life. The opening third of most classic ethnographies is taken up by rapport-building processes. However, the time needed for classic ethnography exceeds the time available for conducting rapid assessment. That is why most of the earlier rapid assessment projects were conducted by veteran ethnographers who were already grounded in the culture being studied and simply refocused their ongoing field work to solve a public health problem.

Logistics Problems

Inadequate resources (people's time as well as dollars), and missing or incomplete support infrastructure (administrative support, transcription services) are other common sources of design failure in rapid assessment projects. This is in addition to the problem of not budgeting adequate time to complete tasks at the appropriate level. Time has to be given to rethink analyses, re-do observations and to follow unanticipated leads. Rapid assessment is not like following step-by-step laboratory procedures.

Poor Analysis

Many earlier rapid assessment programs emphasized data collection over qualitative data analysis. This left local groups with massive amounts of well-collected data that they did not know how to analyze; the result was that they could not complete their project. Until recently, public health professionals had little training in qualitative analysis and the literature on qualitative research was also limited when contrasted with publications on quantitative research. Recent publications have made it easier to train individuals to do qualitative research and therefore to conduct rapid assessment projects.

Problems Producing Recommendations and Action Plans

The final task of the field team is the translation of project findings into concrete recommendations. It is critical for the teams to understand that: 1) recommendations are useless if they cannot be acted upon easily; 2) recommendations flow directly from, and must be tied to, specific research findings; 3) recommendations must be achievable in the short run by entities that have buy-in and can influence outcomes; and 4) the number of recommendations should be limited so that stakeholders are not overwhelmed, and recommendations are not trivialized.

There have been cases where research was well done and the data was properly analyzed, but recommendations and action plans were never produced. The failure in these cases was on the part of the embedded community political process that projects seek to influence. Community participation in rapid assessment is a two-edged sword. On the one hand, it is both unethical and virtually impossible to conduct research in communities without a reasonable level of political participation and buy-in. Care must be taken to provide community input at this stage (like the initial stage). However, it should not produce recommendations or calls for action that reflect the concerns and political needs of the community that cannot be tied directly to rapid assessment findings.

Conclusions

This chapter has provided an overview of rapid assessment, and the contexts within which it is done well and effectively. The chapters in this book illustrate the effective use of the method and its potential to inform more effective

This chapter has provided an overview of rapid assessment, and the contexts within which it is done well and effectively. The chapters in this book illustrate the effective use of the method and its potential to inform more effective HIV/AIDS prevention. The most comprehensive review of the application of rapid assessment to drug and HIV-related research was undertaken by the World Health Organization (Fitch and Stimpson 1993). Their report demonstrates both the success and failures of rapid assessment globally. Rapid assessment proved to be more valuable in finding HIV risk conditions and contexts, than had normal surveillance and epidemiological efforts. It is a method for spotting emerging conditions that are not yet visible in other data sets. It also has the potential for developing interventions that fix the social and cultural context of risk-takers. In addition, rapid assessment is designed to shorten the gap between research for specific programmatic purposes and the implementation of sound intervention strategies that are effective in the cultural and day-to-day world of those at risk (Fitch and Stimpson 2003; Scrimshaw et al. 1992; Trotter and Needle 2001).

Finally, it is of equal importance to the science that rapid assessment makes it possible for communities to have control over their own research "destinies." Properly used, rapid assessment methods can help address the resistance to participating in public health programs encountered in racial and ethnic minority communities in the United States and elsewhere (Singer 1993; Singer and Weeks 2004). Distrust is an appropriate response from communities of color to the ethical failures of earlier research in their communities. For example, the infamous Tuskegee Syphilis Study is remembered, in which syphilis infections were left untreated for over twenty years, as is the inaccurate stigmatizing and labeling of Haitians as a particularly virulent HIV risk group in a 1983–1984 study. These abuses in public health are not easily forgotten.

References

Almedon A.M., Blumenthal, U., Manderson, L. (1997) *Hygiene Evaluation Procedures: Approaches for Assessing Water and Sanitation-related Hygiene Practices*. Boston: International Nutrition Foundation for Developing Countries.

Askew, I., Tapsoba, P., Ouedraogo, Y., et al. (1993) "Quality of Care in Family Planning Programmes: A Rapid Assessment in Burkina Faso." *Health Policy and Planning* 8 (1): 19–32.

Ayepong, I.A., Bertha, A., Dzikunu, H., et al. (1995) *The Malaria Manual*. Geneva: World Health Organization.

Bentley M.E., Pelto, G.H., Straus, W.L., et al. (1988) "Rapid Ethnographic Assessment: Applications in a Diarrhea Management Program." *Social Science and Medicine.* 27 (1):107–116.

Bernard, H. Russell (Ed.) (1998) *Handbook of Methods in Cultural Anthropology*. Walnut Creek: Altamira Press.

Braunstein, M.S. (1993) "Sampling a Hidden Population: Noninstitutionalized Drug Users AIDS." *Education and Prevention* 5 (2): 131–140.

Dale, J., Shipman, C., Lacock, L., Davies, M. (1996) "Creating a Shared Vision of Out-of-Hours Care: Using Rapid Appraisal Methods to Create an Inter-agency, Community Oriented Approach to Service Development." *BMJ* 312 (7040): 1206–1210.

Fitch, Chris, Stimpson, G.V. (2003) *RAR-Review: An International Review of Rapid Assessments Conducted on Drug Use*. Geneva: Department of Mental Health and Substance Abuse, World Health Organization.

Griffiths, P., Gossop, M., Powis, B., Strang, J. (1993) "Reaching Hidden Populations of Drug Users by Privileged Access Interviewers: Methodological and Practical Issues." *Addiction* 88 (12): 1617–1626.

Heaver, R. (1991) *Participative Rural Appraisal. Potential Applications to Family Planning, Health and Nutrition Programs*. Washington, DC: Technical Department Asia Region World Bank.

Johnson, J.C. (1990) *Selecting Ethnographic Informants*. Newbury Park, CA: Sage Publications.

Kuzel, Anton J. (1992) Sampling in Qualitative Inquiry. In Benjamin F. Crabtree and William L. Miller (eds) *Doing Qualitative Research*. Research Methods for Primary Care, Vol. 3, (pp. 31–44). Newbury Park, CA: Sage Publications.

Lee, T., Price, M. (1995) "Indicators and Research Methods for Rapid Assessment of a Tuberculosis Control Programme. Case Study of a Rural Area in South Africa." *Tubercle. Lung. Dis*. 76 (5): 1002–1010.

Lubrosky, Mark R., Rubinstein, R.L. (1995) "Sampling in Qualitative Research: Rationale, Issues and Methods." *Research on Aging* Vol. 17 (1): 89–113.

Malilay, J., Flanders, W.D., Brogan, D.A. (1997) "Modified Cluster Sampling Method for the Rapid Assessment of Needs after a Disaster; Metodo modificado de muestreo por conglomerados para la evaluacion rapida de necesidades despues de un desastre." *Revista Panamericana de Salud Publica/ Pan-American Journal of Public Health* 2 (1): 7–12.

Materia, E., Imoka, G., Berhe, C. et al. (1995) "Rapid Surveys in Support of District Health Information Systems: an Experience from Uganda." *East African Medical Journal* 72 (1): 15–18.

Miller, A.C., Payne, B.S. (1993) "Qualitative Versus Quantitative Sampling to Evaluate Population and Community Characteristics at a Large River Mussel Bed." *Am. Midl. Nat*. 130 (1): 133–145.

Needle, R.H., Trotter, R.T., II, Goosby, E., et al. (2000) "Methodologically Sound Rapid Assessment and Response: Providing Timely Data for Policy Development on Drug Use Interventions and HIV Prevention." *International Journal of Drug Policy* 11: 19–23.

Nickel, Bettina, Berger, M., Schmidt, P., Plies, K. (1995) "Qualitative Sampling in a Multi-method Survey: Practical Problems of Method Triangulation in Sexual Behavior Research." Quality and Quantity 29 (3): 223–240.

Parry, Charles D.H., Quarriasha Adool Karim, M.S. (1999) Country Report for South Africa, Global Research Network Meeting on HIV Prevention in Drug-Using Populations Second Annual Meeting Report. August 26–28, Atlanta, Georgia: National Institute on Drug Abuse National Institutes of Health.

Rhodes T., Stimson G.V., Fitch F., et al. (1999) "Rapid Assessment, Injecting Drug Use, and Public Health." *Lancet* 354: 65–68.

Schensul, J.J., LeCompte, M.D. (1999) *Ethnographer's Toolkit*. Walnut Creek, CA: Altamira Press.

Scrimshaw S., Carballo M., Ramos L., Blair B.A. (1991) "The AIDS Rapid Anthropological Assessment Procedures: a tool for health education planning and evaluation." *Health Education Quarterly* 18: 111–123.

Scrimshaw, S.M., Hurtado E. (1987) *Rapid Assessment Procedures for Nutrition and Primary Health Care: Anthropological Approaches to Improving Programme Effectiveness*. Los Angeles: University of California Latin American Center Publications, References Series, Vol. 11.

Scrimshaw S., Nevin S., Gleason G.R. (eds.) (1992) *Rapid Assessment Procedures Qualitative Methodologies for Planning and Evaluation of Health Related Programs*. Boston: International Nutrition Foundation for Developing Countries.

Singer, Merrill (1999) Studying Hidden and Hard-to-Research Populations. In J. Schensul, M. LeCompte, R. Trotter, E. Cromley and M. Singer (eds.) *The Ethnographer's Toolkit*. (pp.164–241). Walnut Creek, CA: Altamira Press.

Singer, Merrill (1993) "Knowledge for Use: Anthropology and Community-Centered Substance Abuse Research." *Social Science and Medicine* 37 (1): 15–26.

Singer, Merrill (2000) "Evaluating a National AIDS Study." *Society for Applied Anthropology Newsletter* 11 (3): 3–5.

Singer, Merrill and Weeks, M. (2004) The Hartford Model of AIDS Practice/Research Collaboration. In Ed Trickett, (ed.) *Community Intervention and HIV/AIDS: Affecting the Community Context*. (pp. 153–175) Oxford: Oxford University Press.

Stimson G.V., Fitch, C., Rhodes, T., Ball A. (1999) "Rapid Assessment and Response: Methods for Developing Public Health Responses to Drug Problems." *Drug and Alcohol Review* 18: 317–325.

Sudman, Seymour, Kalton, G.N. (1986) "Developments in the Sampling of Special Populations." *Annual Review of Sociology* 12: 401–429.

Sudman, Seymour, Sirken, M.G., Cowan, C.D. (1988) Sampling Rare and Elusive Populations. *Science* 240 (4855): 991–996.

Trotter, Robert T., II (1997) "Anthropological Midrange Theories in Mental Health Research: Selected Theories, Methods, and Systematic Approaches to At-Risk Populations." *Ethos* 25 (2): 259–274.

Trotter, Robert T., II, Schenshul, J.J. (1998) Methods in Applied Anthropology. In H. Russell Bernard (ed.) *Handbook of Methods in Cultural Anthropology* (pp. 691–736). Walnut Creek, CA: Altamira Press.

Trotter, II, R.T., Needle R.H. (1999) Crisis Response Teams and Communities Combat HIV/AIDS in Racial and Ethnic Minority Populations: Rapid Assessment, Rapid Response, and Evaluation Field Assessment Training Workbook. Washington: Office of HIV/AIDS Policy, Department of Health and Human Services.

Trotter, II, Robert T., Bedirhan U., Chatterji, S., et al. (2001) Cross-Cultural Applicability Research on Disablement: Models and Methods for the Revision of an International Classification. *Human Organization* 60 (1): 13–27.

Van Meter, Karl M. (1990) Sampling and Cross-Classification Analysis in International Social Research. In Oyen, Else (ed.) *Comparative methodology: Theory and Practice in International Social Research.* Sage Studies in International Sociology, Vol. 40. (pp. 172–186). London: Sage Publications.

Watters, John K.; Biernacki, P. (1989) Targeted Sampling: Options for the Study of Hidden Populations. *Social Problems* 36 (4): 416–430.

World Health Organization (1998) *Rapid Assessment and Response Guide on Injecting Drug Use*. Geneva: World Health Organization.

World Health Organization and United Nations Joint Programme on HIV/AIDS (1998) *The Rapid Assessment and Response Guide on Substance Use and Sexual Risk Behavior*. Geneva: WHO and UNAIDS.

Whyte, William Foote (1995) Encounters with Participatory Action Research, *Qualitative Sociology* 18 (3): 289–299.

Notes

1. Cultural domains are coherent areas of culture that need to be explored, such as drug use, the environment, risks, etc.

2. The population segments may be different lifestyle groups such as policy makers, health providers and IDUs who have different views of drug use, or they may be groups with contrasting experiences (such as men and women, youth and adults, etc.). These segments have to be determined for each project.

Chapter 3

Responding to the AIDS Crisis in Newark, New Jersey

Ric Curtis
Alix Conde
Maria Irizarry
Christina Wolf

Prelude to the AIDS Epidemic

De-industrialization was well advanced in Newark by the 1960s. Entire industries either moved or went out of business and laid-off thousands of workers. Breweries, tanneries, and large corporations, such as General Electric and Westinghouse, closed plants and moved offices. Unemployment in Newark was triple the national average. The hardest hit sector of the workforce was African Americans who also experienced political powerlessness, lack of affordable housing and police brutality. African Americans were fed up by the summer of 1967. Five days of rioting, from July 12th–17th marked the city's economic and social collapse. Twenty-three people were killed and over one thousand were injured, leaving between $10 million and $15 million in damaged property. Apart from the visible damage, the riots also devastated the city's community life.

The riot was triggered by black residents' grievances against police brutality and, specifically the beating and arrest of an African American cab driver, John Smith, by white officers. In the riot, black residents' grievances against white-run businesses led to arson, looting and major property damage. The aggressive police response to the looting only increased violence and racism against African Americans. The police and National Guard were responsible for 80% of the fatalities. After the riots, the chaos, and administrative instability, much of the city's white middle class fled, leaving the remaining population without a tax-base for essential services. Deindustrialization and racial discrimination in Newark proved a lethal combination, especially for poorly educated young blacks trying to enter the job market. It was under these conditions that Newark's streets exploded. Soon afterward, illicit drugs appeared and began an almost forty-year reign to the present over minority youth, a group that is even more alienated, poverty stricken, and disillusioned than the 1967 rioters (Herman 2002). It is no coincidence that HIV/AIDS would be epidemic in the very same communities and with the same population that rioted in the 1960s, and has yet to recover. Like a deadly shadow, AIDS follows poverty and the loss of hope, a Grim Reaper of the noxious consequences of intense social suffering.

AIDS in Newark

By 1999, Newark had the unenviable distinction of ranking 6th in the nation with respect to the number of AIDS cases (CDC 1999) when compared with other large cities. The disease has ravaged the African American community, whose members make up more than 80% of the reported cases in the city and 20% of all AIDS cases in the state of New Jersey (Newark OHHS 1999).

The New Jersey Department of Health and Human Services estimates that more than 60% of the AIDS cases have been among heterosexual injecting drug users (IDUs), but the proportion of cases attributable to injecting drug use is almost certainly higher than this. It cannot be more accurately estimated because the source of infection for the significant number of homosexual IDUs with AIDS cannot be reliably attributed to a single factor. The bottom line is this: there is an epidemic of HIV/AIDS in Newark whose progression surpasses every other city in the state and most others in the nation. The epidemic has disproportionately affected the African American community, primarily through injecting drug use. Perhaps most alarming is that other major cities like New York, Miami, and San Francisco made progress in 1998–1999 in reducing the rate of reported AIDS cases, but Newark continued to worsen from 44.6% (per 100,000 population) to 47% over the course of only one year (CDC 1999).

One bright spot in an otherwise fairly bleak picture of public health in Newark is that the greatest decrease in the number of deaths in the late 1990s has been in the category of HIV infection, especially among the population of 25–44 years and older. The trend in newly diagnosed AIDS cases continues to decline as well. Still, AIDS remains the leading cause of death of Newark residents 25–44 years of age, accounting for nearly half of all deaths. Furthermore, the gains in this area are more likely the outcome of advances in the medical treatment of the disease rather than changes in local approaches to fighting the epidemic (Newark OHHS 1999, 123).

One major impediment to effectively addressing the HIV/AIDS epidemic in Newark has been the city's dire economic climate. For many people, the more immediate needs of food, shelter and employment continue to overshadow HIV/AIDS as priorities in their daily lives. Only over the last several years has there finally been evidence that Newark is beginning to recover from the riots that devastated the city more than thirty years ago, but many areas of the beleaguered city have yet to benefit from these improvements. In addition, many Newark residents hold the view that the "new" Newark of recently constructed homes and impressive civic improvements offers evidence of an increasingly split city, one part focused on the future, the other mired in the poverty of the past.

The Team and Local Strategy

In order to more proactively respond to its AIDS epidemic, the Newark City Council declared a public health emergency in 1999. The Congressional Black Caucus had secured funds to fight AIDS and the U.S. Department of Health and Human Services (DHHS) had made some of these funds available for technical assistance through a Crisis Response Team (CRT). Through consultations between public health officials in Newark and the CRT, a Community Work Group was selected in the Spring of 2000 to advise and guide the Newark RARE Field Research Team that was subsequently chosen from a pool of local residents.

The Newark Field Research Team was composed of individuals who were nominated by members of the Community Work Group. Beginning in July 2000, potential members received three days of intensive training from the CRT in RARE methods and techniques to collect and analyze data. Following this training period, senior personnel at DHHS in consultation with the CRT, reviewed the strengths and weaknesses of the nominees and selected fifteen of them to comprise the Field Research Team. The team was initially composed of six women and nine men, who ranged in age from seventeen to more than sixty, but over the course of ten weeks (7/12–9/20) of data collection, several members of the team dropped out and a few others were added.

The data collection efforts of the Field Research Team were continuously monitored by members of the Newark Department of Health and Human Services and two ethnographers selected by the CRT. When a local ethnographer could not be found, the CRT recruited Ric Curtis and Alix Conde from New York City. The CRT and Newark officials were concerned that Curtis and Conde's lack of knowledge about Newark and its people might be an impediment to producing an informed and comprehensive picture of the AIDS epidemic in the city. In retrospect, however, it was precisely their lack of knowledge about Newark that made the data collection process and subsequent analysis more impartial than that of a local ethnographer who might have had preconceived notions about the city.

The first political issue we had to address as Field Team members was not to give the appearance of political favoritism in the places around the city where we conducted the study. The Field Research Team was directed to divide their work evenly among five wards—North, South, East, West, and Central. At first this seemed problematic because other RARE cities had found that high-risk activities were often concentrated in socio-geographic hot spots. Initially we assumed this was the same in Newark. Next, the CRT in consultation with its local partners identified the at-risk populations to be targeted by the Team. Initially, the at-risk populations included male and female sexworkers, drug injectors, MSMs (men who have sex with men), and WSWs (women who have sex with women). As the research process proceeded we identified additional risk groups in our weekly debriefing sessions. For example, there were at least two types of female sex workers: those who worked for themselves and those who were "managed" by pimps. The daily routines of these two groups of sex worker differed considerably, a fact that had important implications for effective outreach efforts. Also engaged in high-risk behaviors were sexually active youths, senior citizens and immigrant groups, especially Central Americans, Haitians and Africans.

Data collection began on July 17, 2000, with direct observation. Over the next ten weeks more than 637 hours of observations were made in various selected locales in the targeted wards and thirty-nine individuals recruited from these sites were interviewed. Ten focus groups were held at the health department and other agency offices, and in the apartments of study participants; one of our interview sites doubled as a shooting gallery/crack house. The focus groups were designed to capture a wide variety of voices and perspectives on the HIV/AIDS epidemic in Newark. Three were done with public and private agency "service providers." The most difficult focus groups to convene were of "community leaders." Focus groups also were held with HIV positive persons, Latino youths, MSMs, WSWs, and hard-core drug users. There were no focus groups composed exclusively of injecting drug users or sex workers, but individuals in these risk categories were well represented in other focus groups.

Findings

Where are Drugs Used?

Observations, interviews and focus groups confirmed that high-risk activities regularly occurred in each of the hot spots that were selected, but ongoing analysis of the data during weekly debriefing sessions suggested that focusing on the "geography of risk" was misleading. Drug use was diffused in such a manner as to render the idea of a hot spot almost meaningless; other investigators studying crime found the same dispersal of sites (George Kelling, Personal Communication). The idea of hot spots began to lose its appeal and other ways of conceptualizing the problem emerged as a better fit.

Hard drug users (heroin and cocaine) were dispersed all over Newark and individuals reported in interviews that they preferred to use drugs in the privacy of their own homes; but other places were used as well. In a focus group with hard drug users the reported site of their "last injection" was telling: one said, "I injected about an hour ago between two schools." A second replied, "I shot up about half an hour ago on the street behind a tree." A third participant recounted how she shielded herself within a crowd of friends to inject herself with a dosage of heroin right on the sidewalk, in broad daylight. Another said that her "wake up" that morning [first injection of the day] was done "in the bathroom at the courthouse," where she had to appear for a hearing.

In general, most people agreed that public drug use was considerably more discreet than had been the case in earlier years. There was increasing stigmatization and the police were more aggressive. Another factor that has pushed public drug use into less visible places is the urban renewal that is now evident in several parts of Newark. Several homeless hard drug users said that they used to spend much of their time in downtown Newark, near Penn station, but that several urban renewal projects, like the NJPAC Center, have forced them to relocate their drug use activities. One homeless injector complained that the removal of benches made the public parks in downtown Newark less attractive to sleep in and use drugs. He and others have begun to live at and use drugs in isolated places like "the trailers" (near Raymond Blvd. and Freeman St.), a storage yard for empty tractor-trailer cargo containers.

A friend's house was the next most favored place to use drugs. Of course, the expectation in these circumstances is that the drugs will be shared. As one injector explained, "As long as I give her a taste [some of the drugs], I'm welcome to use the place." Many hard drug users spoke about the many "houses" in Newark that specialize in providing space for people to use drugs. As one female Puerto Rican injector explained:

> There's quite a few houses like that in the area. There's at least three of those houses nearby where I cop [buy drugs]. To go there, I have to give the owner at least a ten [CCs] . . . almost half of the bag. The people who run these houses are either Puerto Ricans or Blacks.

The seeming ubiquity of these "houses" throughout Newark reflects the diffuse character of local drug markets. Drug-using spots seem equally dispersed throughout the city. But despite the drug use across much of Newark, very specific people used drugs.

Who Are the Hard Drug Users?

Poly-drug Users

The most important similarity linking members of the various groups that were observed (including service provider groups) was the ubiquity of poly-drug use. There can be no doubt that the AIDS epidemic in Newark is driven by drug use, especially when those drugs are injected. With the exception of the focus groups conducted with Latino youths and community leaders, every focus group that the Field Research Team convened was dominated by people who were current or ex-poly-drug users. The overwhelming presence of poly-drug users at almost every step of the data collection process led the Team to more carefully examine linkages between the different poly-drug using subgroups as a potential route for the transmission of the AIDS virus.

Based upon a statistical profile of the AIDS epidemic in Newark, our examination began with the person most likely to get infected with HIV; African American male drug injectors. We found no reason to question this profile. But we did find some important additional dimensions. One important finding is that most people were poly-drug users who consumed drugs in a variety of ways other than by injection. Several hard drug users claimed that they were not injectors, but were, nevertheless, HIV-positive. For example, in the "women who have sex with women" (WSWs) focus group, one participant, a middle-aged African American woman who lives with her twenty-five year old daughter said:

> I'm HIV positive and I smoke cocaine. I've been smoking it for ten to twelve years. I've never really tried to stop. I like it. I only stopped once—for six years—when I went down South. When I returned to Newark in 1996, I started again. I found out that I was HIV positive in 1996 when I had a tubal pregnancy and they tested me when I went to take care of that in the hospital.

Many HIV-positive research subjects claimed that they had never injected drugs, but admitted to hard drug use and to intimate and frequent interactions with people who did inject drugs. It was clear to the Team that the appropriate category of HIV risk should encompass more than simply injectors. Clearly, the research subjects saw it this way. As one of them, a forty-one-year-old African American male, noted:

> I'm a heroin user. I sniff about two bags a day. I've never injected it, but I've never been tested for HIV either. I don't want to know my HIV status. So many of my friends have it, I'm afraid of finding out.

Not Young People

Most of the hard drug users who were observed or interviewed were over thirty years of age. Indeed, the most promising development in Newark has been the growing generational divide in drug use. With few exceptions, young people in Newark avoid using hard drugs and view those who do with contempt. As one forty-year-old Puerto Rican female drug injector noted:

> [The young drug dealers] only smoke weed. The majority don't even do that, smoke or drink. They just want the moolah [money]. There's a certain spot where there's a guy who sells who is very disrespectful to us. He curses at them, 'mira, maricon, pendejo [Spanish explicatives] . . .' He's about nineteen years old.

Senior Citizens

If the good news is that young people are being turned off to hard drugs, the bad news is that older people, both middle-aged and senior citizens continue to be drawn to them. As evidence of how problematic the rash of senior citizen drug use has become, one service provider during a focus group instructed the ethnographers to visit the check cashing establishments that day. They saw female sex workers waiting outside for elderly men to exit after having cashed their monthly Social Security checks. Bored and lonely, these elderly men were paying for sex, and in the process, developing serious drug habits and contracting HIV. The increasing stigma attached to heroin and crack use makes no difference. For example, one new injector, a forty-five-year-old African American woman, commented on her own worsening pattern of drug use:

> I've been skin popping dope for two years now, but smoking cocaine is my drug of choice. The way I started smoking coke is through friends who told me that they 'fell in love' with smoking cocaine. I had to try it.

Circle of Well-Known Partners

As this woman suggests, in Newark, there is a strong connection between an individual's pattern of drug use and their network of friendships and other relationships. Overwhelmingly, the evidence suggests that people use drugs within a circle of well-known peers. But the occasional mention of outsiders suggests that the many small networks of hard drug-using groups form a large, interconnected web of users that can be traced well beyond the borders of Newark. One Latina drug injector, for example, talked about the "white heroin users" that she used drugs with and bought drugs for on a daily basis:

> They [white heroin users] come from all over. Some come from Perth Amboy. About ten people come [to me] everyday. They're regular customers. If I'm not around, they'll look for someone else who I introduced them to that they could trust. They come to buy bundles and bricks [bundle=10 bags of heroin; brick=10 bundles]. They don't take my word that the stuff is good, they try it out. They shoot it behind the McDonalds where I take them. That's my favorite place.

White Users in Newark

The people we interviewed said that whites buy most of the drugs in Newark rather than local users and their presence among users is greater than most people think. For example, one focus group (of WSWs) included a twenty-one year-old homeless white girl who, of late, spends most of her time in Newark.

> I mainly use heroin [inject], but I use lots of other stuff too: coke, which I sometimes shoot or smoke, Ecstasy, Ketamine . . . lots of stuff. I get money mostly from panhandling, but I also clean houses and sometimes I dance in Atlantic City. I don't strip, I dance in a bikini. I'll make about

> $200 from a night of dancing. With that money, I'll usually buy a bundle of dope and use the rest for my other expenses.

As young whites, largely from suburban communities, continue to experiment with heroin (and they continue to be the only type of young people who show any interest in the drug whatsoever), there is evidence that many of them are spending considerable amounts of time in Newark. One reason that their presence has gone largely undetected is that they are spending time in places where they are less likely to encounter outreach workers, health care professionals or the police. For example, on one occasion, the ethnographers walked along the railroad tracks near the Broadway Townhouses. Over less than one city block along the tracks (a place they were warned to avoid because it was too "dangerous"), the ethnographers observed eight hard drug users injecting in the shadows of the bushes; half of them were white. While comparatively few Newark residents seem to share drugs with people outside their networks of friends and acquaintances, in private locales like houses or apartments, and in public spaces like parks and abandoned buildings, a much broader array of hard drug users is commonly found.

Immigrant Starters?

The Field Research Team observed mainly African American and Puerto Rican hard drug users, but there was some evidence that other nationalities may be involved in hard drug use as well. For example, the Team spoke with several heroin users and local residents who told them about the heavy presence of Haitians in the area. Another group which had a visible presence on the street and was reputed to be involved with hard drug distribution, and perhaps use, was "Africans." While the Team was not able to confirm whether Haitians or "Africans" are involved in hard drug use or distribution, their presence suggests that they may be placing themselves at risk for HIV. Observations in Latino neighborhoods also suggest that the influx of Central Americans over the last decade, including many Mexicans, may bring another layer of hard drug users to Newark. More information is needed regarding these ethnic sub-groups to assess the degree to which they are, or are not, involved with hard drugs.

What Are They Doing?

The overwhelming number of hard drug users who were interviewed or observed were poly-drug users who had been using drugs for many years. As such, most of them had developed routines that were quite predictable, but they often admitted that their drug-using careers were characterized by earlier periods of bingeing, replete with a range of risky behaviors. For example, one newly employed hard drug user who had settled into a weekly routine of use, noted, "I started smoking cocaine over the last ten years. At the height of my use, I was having a smoke-fest every day."

For many, careers in drug use brought them through several distinct phases, often concluding with more moderate patterns of use or complete abstinence. One user in an MSM focus group proudly stated:

> I started doing drugs at twenty-four years old, late for most, when I saw coke for the first time. My drug of choice eventually became dope [heroin], which I sniffed. I never injected it. I'm now on a methadone detox program. I started at 75mg and I'm down to forty. I also used to use "sticks" [Xanex]. A doctor gave me a prescription for it to help me sleep, but I started using them for enjoyment.

The development of predictable drug-using routines among long-time users does not necessarily mean that they use drugs with greater care. Indeed, there is ample evidence to suggest that many hard drug users continue to engage in high-risk practices. While members of the Field Research Team were unable to directly observe injection events while collecting data, several pieces of evidence suggest that widespread sharing of potentially contaminated injection equipment occurs on a regular basis. When injectors in one focus group were asked how long they re-use a syringe before buying another, one participant replied "until the numbers [on the barrel] wear off." Clearly, injection equipment is being used again and again, until it wears out. It is possible that injectors are cleaning their injection with bleach or some other cleansing agent, but observations throughout Newark revealed a complete lack of harm-reduction materials of any kind and not a single injector said that they ever systematically cleaned their syringes.

Sometimes, it is not what you see; it is what you do not see that signals danger. In the case of drug injectors in Newark, the almost complete absence of discarded injection paraphernalia in the streets and near drug-using locales speaks to the degree to which that equipment is being hoarded and re-used by injectors. It was not simply the absence of discarded syringes that was striking, but the invisibility of all other pieces of the injectors' ensemble. The absence of discarded "cookers" (bottle caps in which injectors heat their solution before drawing it into a syringe) indicates the degree to which "cooking" drugs (which is done, in part, to help remove impurities) has been replaced by "cold shaking" the drug (i.e., simply adding water); this is a process which many drug users feel results in health problems like abscesses. The absence of cotton filters through which the solution is drawn to filter out impurities was also alarming. Some injectors said that they no longer filter the drug, while at least one injector had an even more surprising story:

> I used to throw my cotton away, but lately, I've been saving them in a jar for my friend. When he's dope sick, I'll give them to him. He adds water to the cotton, squeezes it out and is able to get a G-shot from it [to stave off withdrawal].

The absence of any evidence that harm-reduction materials among hard drug users, especially injectors, suggests many have not altered their behavior to protect themselves from HIV despite their knowledge about the epidemic. Most injectors insist that they do not share drugs in risky ways. They do admit to sharing drugs but only with their intimate partners. There appears to be a big discrepancy between their words and deeds.

When Are They Doing It?

Early in the data collection process, the Field Research Team realized that hard drug users' risk for contracting HIV was not distributed evenly over the day, week, or month. There were certain times of the day that hard drug users were more likely to engage in risky behaviors when using drugs. For heroin users, the beginning of the day, when people are beginning to feel withdrawal symptoms ("dope sick"), was especially stressful and was often characterized by panicked drug use (i.e., shooting up in the bathroom of the courthouse). For crack smokers, greatest risk often comes near the end of a lengthy episode of use: "When crack-heads are fiending for another hit, they'll do anything for it," explained one user.

In general, however, hard drug users attempted to avoid placing themselves in situations where they were desperate for more drugs. Many heroin users spoke about saving their "wake up" bag from the previous night to ensure that they would not have to scramble around for their drugs in the morning. As noted above, many hard drug users had well-developed and predictable routines. One female poly-drug user who had developed a consistent pattern of use explained: "Between my monthly check and my man's weekly salary, I never have a problem getting straight [in the morning]." Another said that she is able to plan in advance for the next morning, but should something unexpected happen, "When I'm dope sick, I have one or two people who will look after me."

Though there was evidence that most hard drug users attempted to organize their drug taking in ways that were predictable, there was still considerable variation in the daily patterns that members of the Field Research Team observed and heard about. The many variations were not merely idiosyncratic patterns disconnected from each other. The hard drug users were connected in myriad ways (by kinship, culture, business, etc.) and so were their drug use routines. Our observations have convinced us that when they used drugs (time of day and time of month) and risk behaviors are related, and furthermore, that monthly patterns of drug use are perhaps the most important ones to consider when assessing HIV risk among hard drug users.

Many hard drug users noted that their patterns of drug use were dependent upon checks they received at the beginning of each month. The first week of each month was always characterized by greater drug use, including bingeing. The latter half of the month was always characterized by less drug use, more "hustling," and a greater likelihood of sharing drugs with others. One female injector summed up the difference between the first week and the remainder of each month:

> At the first of the month, everyone has money. By the fifteenth, you have to go out there and struggle to get your money for your "wake up." Sometimes, you have to do what you have to do. You have to prostitute out there to get your money. And after you get your money, you got to go to the spot and cop your stuff. And sometimes, they don't got the needles. Sometimes the man's not there to buy the needles. You go to the other one, and the other one ain't got it. Sometimes, there ain't no needles out here, put it this way. In the first of the month, it's not as bad as the middle of the month.

A female focus group participant put it even more succinctly: "Women from the projects get high from the first to the fifth. After that, they go ho'ing [whoring] for the rest of the month." Nearly everyone agreed that after the first week of each month, many hard drug users must combine resources with others to sustain a drug habit.

There are many hard drug users who do not receive a monthly check and who have to "hustle" every day to secure their drugs. But even these drug users noted that their drug use was affected by those who did rely on monthly payments.

Outreach to At-Risk People

Outreach to people at-risk for HIV is a critical component of any attempt to prevent disease transmission. Though there is, apparently, a considerable amount of funding for HIV-related outreach programs in Newark, there was an alarming lack of visible or effective outreach being done in the city, especially to sex workers and drug injectors. In the many observations and interviews conducted throughout the city, there was no apparent evidence of any outreach activities of any kind. No typical outreach materials—like condoms, literature, or bleach kits—were observed to be in the possession of at-risk people by any members of the Field Research Team. Even worse, when asked, people had never seen outreach conducted in their neighborhoods or in the places where they engage in risky behaviors such as commercial sex strolls, shooting galleries or crack houses). One female drug injector said:

> No one ever goes to the "houses" [where people go to inject drugs] to offer the [HIV] test. In the times that I've ever been there, I've never seen anyone go behind the McDonalds to offer anything either. I don't think they even know about that spot.

When the ethnographers accompanied members of the Field Research Team to sites where risky behaviors were obviously taking place, people were asked if they had ever seen outreach workers in the area. Several Latina sex workers greedily shoved dozens of condoms that we had brought into their pockets as they gave us a quizzical look. We had, after all, asked a stupid question: no, they had never seen such a thing. The irony of this scene was that, in the background, the ethnographers observed a Community Health Center. When one of the sex workers was asked about the Health Center, she said, "Oh yeah, if I ever get real sick, I'll go there." Clearly, however, she didn't have much of a relationship with any health care providers there, despite the fact that she solicits business and smokes crack virtually on their doorstep.

When the ethnographers visited "the trailers," the hard drug users who were encountered there examined the bleach kits that the Team brought with them very carefully: apparently, they had never seen one. When asked, they responded that they had never seen an outreach worker of any kind come to "the trailers." The story was the same in every single place that field observations were conducted by the Field Research Team, with one caveat. Some at-risk people and service providers talked about "the big vans that come around." Some of the vans, they said, offer HIV testing while others offer food, clothing and referrals to indigent people. While many people said that the services that these vans offered were important, they were also critical of them. One participant of an HIV-positive focus group complained: "[there are] people who come around in a van, but they don't go into the streets. And many people don't want the clothes that they offer. Those who do take the clothes, take them to sell later."

While service providers and community leaders all agreed that outreach was an important component of HIV prevention, there seemed to be a fundamental lack of knowledge and of training in effective outreach. What outreach they had was restricted to small and overworked geographic areas where people had grown tired of the "message." In Newark, there was a palpable fear of going to other areas where the highest risk behaviors were taking place. This fear did not seem to be based on experience. No outreach worker reported any incident where their workers were harmed in the course of doing their job.

It is our view that their fear was based on myth and misinformation, and was an outcome of poor training and planning and performance expectations. One vignette illustrates this point: The ethnographers were repeatedly warned to "avoid the railroad tracks near the Broadway Townhouses." The image of search parties looking for dead bodies was mentioned several times by several people. With some trepidation, the ethnographers decided to take a look and encountered numerous drug users concealed in the bushes. They proved to be quite receptive to outreach efforts and several asked about referrals to drug treatment. The condoms and bleach kits brought by the ethnographers were greatly appreciated; they were "surprised that anyone cared." They then sought to direct us to other places where we might find people in need. The fact that no outreach occurred here speaks volumes about the lack of a focused and coordinated effort in Newark to combat the epidemic.

Recommendations

The findings presented above suggest that much more needs to be done in Newark if substantial progress is to be made against the HIV/AIDS epidemic. These data could have provided local policy makers and public health officials with great ammunition in their efforts to compete for state and federal resources to combat the epidemic. But the unfortunate reality is that the RARE process was not accompanied by funds for new prevention efforts. So our recommendations are modest and work within existing funding arrangements.

> Recommendation 1: Reinvigorate the culture of AIDS service provision in Newark by addressing the apathy and burnout that afflicts many agencies.

After nearly twenty years of fighting the AIDS epidemic, many health care professionals and social service providers are disillusioned that visible progress against the disease is not evident in Newark. Complaining that there is "no light at the end of the tunnel," many professionals spoke with sadness, frustration and regret that more has not been accomplished and that the experience of working in the field has adversely affected so many of their peers. Many complained that their repetitive jobs offered low salaries, little prestige, few opportunities for advancement, and insufficient training in up-to-date information relevant to their clients.

Many excellent suggestions for improvements were articulated by providers. In their opinions, a centrally coordinated program to which private and public agencies can send their employees should be established and should offer such things as relevant HIV-related trainings, updates on the latest advances in treatment and prevention, and seminars that build professional credentials. Of particular importance are opportunities for employees to attend support groups and receive individual counseling to relieve job-related stress.

> Recommendation 2: Using up-to-date information collected locally, develop on-going training programs for service providers, especially outreach workers, who serve at-risk populations. Minimum standards of training should be required for all service providers, regardless of institutional affiliation.

Many outreach workers, in particular, chafed at the poor quality of training they had received, and, even more so, at the limitations that were placed upon their activities by the various agencies where they worked. For example, some outreach workers were told to avoid certain parts of the city; others were told that they could not carry condoms; still others said that they were instructed not to even talk about safe sex (only abstinence). The point here is that many of the people who are employed to provide services to at-risk populations in Newark are not adequately trained in the theories, methods, and techniques in their field, nor are they given the appropriate tools or support to do so. Increases in the salaries of outreach workers are needed to elevate the prestige of the position and underscore the importance of the work. But still lack of training overshadows all else.

Recommendation 3: Coordinate outreach to at-risk populations: Track and respond to identified patterns of risk.

The evidence collected by the Field Research Team strongly suggests that what little outreach is being done in Newark to at-risk populations is ineffective. A major reason is that the existing teams of outreach workers have settled into daily routines that are based upon outdated assumptions about people's risk behaviors. They have not kept pace with or responded to changes in the patterns of risk exhibited by their target populations. Some outreach workers are aware of "windows of opportunity" for intervention that correspond to the patterns of risk. But this field knowledge is not captured and acted on a systematic manner. The knowledge is important that hard drug users consume more drugs at the beginning of each month, but share with others at a greater rate near the end of each month. Outreach workers could devise more effective ways of promoting less risky drug use based upon this fact.

Serious consideration also needs to be given to providing effective outreach during unusual times and in non-traditional settings. One finding that could benefit from flexibility in outreach is that increasing numbers of senior citizens are spending their Social Security checks on sex and drugs. If this observation is correct, then AIDS-related literature should be available at these check cashing places as well as outreach workers.

A centralized clearinghouse of local information and a centralized coordinating and decision-making body is sorely needed with respect to areas and times of greatest risk. This would ensure the continuous flow of data to inform the activities of outreach workers throughout the city and that all at-risk people and places are attended to.

Recommendation 4: Utilize existing networks of relationships to better access at-risk populations.

Most successful street outreach efforts target geographic locations where risk behaviors are known to take place: drug "copping" areas, shooting galleries, crack houses, commercial sex "strolls," etc. In Newark, most of these indoor locations are not available to the general public; they are accessed through personal connections. Outreach workers should capitalize on these networks of relationships to more easily identify those people who are engaging in behaviors that place them at risk of HIV.

Recommendation 5: Increase the availability and use of harm-reduction materials.

There is a woeful lack of harm-reduction materials of all kinds available to at-risk persons in Newark. Condom distribution needs to be dramatically expanded, especially to commercial sex workers and sexually active youths. Harm-reduction materials need to be made available to injecting drug users. Evidence suggests that those who are at the pinnacle of HIV risk are unlikely to consistently seek out these materials. Thus, it is not enough for harm-reduction materials simply to be made available; these items must be physically put into the hands of those people who need them.

Recommendation 6: Increase HIV testing of underserved populations by coordinating with outreach efforts.

HIV testing programs in Newark reach only a small percentage of those people who should be tested. Each at-risk population discussed in this chapter is unlikely to seek out HIV testing on a routine basis. Efforts should be made through linkages to outreach programs (see above) to recruit more at-risk people, particularly hard drug users, sexually active youths, and truly hidden populations like Haitians, Africans and Central Americans.

Recommendation 7: Increase the variety of social and health services, especially low-threshold services, available to at-risk populations.

Most service providers and at-risk people who the Field Research Team spoke with were extremely critical of the range of social and health services available in Newark. In the area of drug treatment, there was wide agreement that many more treatment slots are needed; but even more importantly, that the city needs programs that offer hope to more than just those people who are ultra-committed to cleaning up their lives. Low-threshold programs, especially drug treatment programs, do not exist in Newark. A reasonable argument could be made that medium-threshold programs are similarly absent. High-threshold, drug-free programs are appropriate and work for some people, but that should not be the only choice available for people who want to move their lives in positive directions.

The appalling lack of harm-reduction services—those that are scientifically proven to be successful in reducing the incidence of HIV/AIDS among at-risk people—is frightening given the amount of time and money that has already been directed at combating this epidemic. It is the kind of egregious oversight that begins to give credence to those who steadfastly maintain that AIDS is a genocidal plot. Serious consideration needs to be given to instituting an entire range of harm-reduction services in Newark, including safe sex programs for commercial sex workers, training in safe injection techniques for injecting drug users and the feasibility of a syringe exchange program.

Report Outcomes

One crucial piece is missing from the RARE report that deserves a book in itself. That is the degree to which the prevention process incrementally builds up from the grassroots rather than being imposed from the top down. It turns out that RARE acted to empower local folks to take ownership of the process and stimulated ongoing dialogue about the findings and recommendations. Even when there was disagreement about recommendations and findings, the report did help identify problems for further exploration and elaboration. It would require local people and resources to do this work and devise solutions. RARE was done locally and was something that Newark residents had largely accomplished by themselves. They recognized that they could do it again when/if the need presented itself. There was no potential for RARE to have any impact without the encouragement, assistance and support of key personnel at the Office of Health and Human Services in Newark and on the HIV Planning Council.

Disbelief

The initial presentations of the RARE findings gave little indication of whether local agencies will act on the recommendations. When the final report was presented to the HIV Planning Council, there was some resistance, a certain level of anger, and distrust of the results as well as the process. Most of this disbelief came from the professionals who saw the report as a critique of their particular services. For example, in the highlighted lack of effective outreach to injection drug users, some service providers responded that existing programs had been overlooked by the researchers. This was a valid concern, but we did not seek to "evaluate" all existing outreach programs in Newark. The RARE process had focused on the vast community of injecting drug users who had not been served by existing programs. Hard drug users continued to be the driving force behind the Newark HIV/AIDS epidemic and it was clear that they had been underserved by existing programs. Thus, RARE underscored the urgent need to refocus energies on the primary vectors of disease transmission.

It was clear that service providers in Newark had worked very hard to create a continuum of care for PLWHA. But the system did not work for everyone who needed treatment, especially those who were at the highest risk of HIV infection. Generally, those people who sought HIV/AIDS services were able to find them and many voiced satisfaction with the quality of care that they received. There were, however, many high-risk persons who refused to seek out existing services (for a variety of reasons) and they presented the greatest challenge to agencies that provide outreach services. RARE revealed disturbing and uncomfortable findings about the most difficult-to-reach HIV-risk populations. This gave agency administrators insight, often for the first time, into how their programs were viewed by the street-level community. This began a wide-ranging discussion about how to change outreach programs to engage and bring these people into the system of care.

An Impact

The report had an impact. The way that outreach services have changed is significant. Hours and routes in outreach have changed and training in outreach has improved. Outreach has now become a critical centerpiece for most of the leading HIV/AIDS programs that operate in Newark. In many cases it has replaced case management as the entry point into the system. This has resulted in a few agencies moving far ahead of others in their ability to bring in previously unserved or underserved clients. These agencies have increased their client populations, the number of services they provide, and consequently, they have been rewarded with significant increases to their budgets.

The RARE process in Newark not only changed outreach services but other HIV services as well. RARE remains the undercurrent for most planning and needs assessment projects in Newark and the surrounding region. A desire to respond to the RARE findings led other types of programs to re-think the way that they deliver services, internally and externally. For example, primary care clinics have recently shifted their hours to accommodate the needs of clients who had avoided the clinic in the past. In addition, dedicated clinics for gays and transgender persons were established in response to their reporting that they were uncomfortable accessing existing services. Ultimately, the impact of RARE on Newark was greater than most of the participants in the process would have predicted. It remains relevant today and stands as testimony to the power of this unique research approach to social problems.

References

Centers for Disease Control and Prevention. (1999) *HIV/AIDS Surveillance Report*, December 31.

Herman, Max. (2002) "Ethnic Succession and Urban Unrest in Newark and Detroit during the Summer of 1967." <http://www.cornwall.rutgers.edu/pdf/Herman-July%202002-Report.pdf>

Newark Office of Health and Human Services. (1999) *Newark Health Profile*.

Chapter 4

AIDS Health Emergency in Chicago

Paul LaKosky
Elijah Ward
Lawrence J. Ouellet

The AIDS Epidemic in Chicago

Over 17,000 AIDS cases have been reported in Chicago. The majority of AIDS diagnoses during the 1980s occurred among non-Hispanic white males who had sex with other men (MSM). This no longer is true. In 1999, African Americans accounted for 68% of new AIDS cases though they constitute only 37% of the city's population. Of the remaining cases, 19% were among non-Hispanic whites and 12% were among Hispanics. The primary mode of HIV transmission also has changed to drug injection. From 1990–1997 the proportion of AIDS cases attributed to sex between men declined from 64% to 41% and the proportion attributed to injection drug use increased from 31% to 43%. This included cases caused by sex with a drug injector or by being born to a mother who injected drugs. Women, especially African American women, account for an increasingly large proportion of HIV infections. Women comprised 23% of AIDS cases diagnosed in 1999, up from 9% in 1990. Among women in Chicago, African Americans constitute 40% of the population but 78% of the AIDS cases diagnosed between 1997 and 1999.

About three-quarters of new AIDS diagnoses continue to occur in persons 30–49 years old. However, high rates of sexually transmitted diseases and pregnancy indicate that many engage in unprotected sex, which places them at risk for HIV infection. Between 1995 and 1997, one hundred twenty-three new AIDS cases were reported among persons 13–24 years old of whom 68% were males. Sixty-seven percent of these cases occurred among non-Hispanic black youth and 23% among Hispanic youth. Sexual contact was the primary risk factor in 72% of these cases (City of Chicago Department of Public Health Epidemiology Program Report, September 1999).

RARE in Chicago

On January 22, 1999, Mayor Richard M. Daley responded to a December 24, 1998 announcement in the Federal Register (67: 247, p. 71290) reporting the availability of Crisis Response Team's (CRT) "to provide multidisciplinary technical assistance teams to localities most highly impacted by HIV/AIDS within racial and ethnic minority communities." A letter from the Mayor, sent to the Director of the Office of HIV/AIDS Policy, initiated the CRT process in Chicago. A positive response to the letter, indicating that Chicago met the criteria for inclusion, came from the U.S. Department of Health and Human Services. Preparations for the implementation of the CRT/RARE project in Chicago began in earnest in August of 2000 with the recruitment of the Community Advisory Committee and Field Assessment Team.

Recruitment of the Community Advisory Committee was conducted during August and September of 2000. Flyers announcing the RARE project were distributed at the HIV/AIDS Prevention Planning Group's monthly meeting, the Ryan White Planning Council's monthly meeting, regional planning group meetings and via a broadcast fax to all Chicago Department of Public Health (CDPH) prevention funded agencies. The Division of STD/HIV/AIDS Public Policy and Programs has a long history of working in partnership with the community in the planning and provision of STD/HIV/AIDS services. Because of this relationship, CDPH was able to draw from a pool of individuals that was both familiar with the unique nature of the HIV/AIDS epidemic in Chicago and representative of the population overall.

Field Assessment Team members were recruited from community-based organizations that received HIV/AIDS prevention funding from CDPH as well as from the community-at-large. Consideration was given to individuals who met the following criteria: 1) previous experience in research and data collection, 2) previous experience with HIV/AIDS outreach programming, 3) access to the desired communities, 4) indigenous to the community, 5) knowledge of the study site, and 6) knowledge of the populations targeted for study. Four teams were organized, each with its own captain who reported to the principal investigator, ethnographer or field administrator. Each team was constructed to include: 1) a racial/cultural mix of members; 2) at least one individual from outside the study area targeted by the team; 3) members with varying experiential backgrounds; 4) an age/gender mix; and 5) several individuals familiar with the site/populations.

Use of the RARE Methods

The four field assessment teams, one per site, began their assessments in November 2000 using four methods common to qualitative research: observation and informal conversations, mapping, formal audio taped interviews and focus groups. These methods were guided by a set of research questions: 1) who are the groups in your area that are at the greatest risk for being or becoming infected with HIV? 2) what are the behaviors and practices that place them at risk?, 3) where do the risks occur? 4) when do the risks occur? 5) why do people engage in these risk practices? and 6) how can risks be avoided or reduced? Interviews with service providers also explored their ability to meet HIV prevention needs and their ideas for improving services. Most of the fieldwork was conducted in November and December of 2000, with some additional work lasting until February 2001.

In observation and informal interviews, field team members typically work in pairs and at different times of the day, night and week. These teams conducted observations in areas where high-risk activities took place or where persons at high risk for HIV infection congregated. Team members consistently spoke with people in these areas, explaining RARE and its goals and asking for insight into current issues affecting their ability to avoid contracting or transmitting HIV infection, or to obtain medical care for HIV infection. These observations and conversations were recorded in field notes that were reviewed by the project ethnographers and discussed in weekly meetings of the entire assessment team.

In mapping, team members drew graphic representations of the geography of current HIV-risk practices and prevention resources in their respective areas. The mapping attempted to include variations according to the time of the day and over a period of a week or month. The field teams conducted formal, audio-taped interviews with persons they selected for their ability to address and provide a range of views regarding the issues of interest. Finally, two focus groups were conducted with injection drug users. Group members were selected by the field teams mainly for their knowledge of drug use scenes, HIV-risk practices and barriers to HIV prevention in their neighborhoods.

The Study Sites

Study sites for the RARE project were selected by the Community Advisory Committee during the October 11, 2000, orientation. In choosing sites, committee members were asked to draw upon their personal and professional knowledge of the HIV/AIDS epidemic in Chicago to identify "hot spots" of HIV/AIDS risk behaviors. Four sites were selected by the committee based on the following criteria: 1) racial/ethnic distribution of populations at each site, 2) geographic distribution of the sites within Chicago, 3) distribution of HIV/AIDS risk factors among sites/populations, and 4) known co-factors for HIV/AIDS at each site. The sites are based upon four of the seventy-seven Chicago study areas:

1. Altgeld Gardens
2. Humboldt Park
3. Cicero Avenue Corridor
4. The Hangout

Given the direction that the AIDS epidemic is going in Chicago, this report will focus on three of the four sites. For a review of findings and recommendations on the Hangout, see http://www.aidschicago.org/pdf/rarereport.pdf.

Altgeld Gardens

"The Gardens," as it is called by those who live there, is located in the Riverdale community. It is on Chicago's far south side and built between 1943 and 1945 in "one of the neighborhoods with the city's highest concentration of subsidized housing" (*Chicago Tribune* 02/21/82). Altgeld Gardens was constructed in a geographically isolated section of Chicago's Far South Side following the city's unofficial but widely acknowledged policy of racial segregation (Shore, 1995).

At the time of its construction, Altgeld Gardens was the largest and most complex housing development of its type in Chicago. It covered nearly 160 acres and was a self-contained small community. In addition to housing, it sported a health station, public library, nursery, clubroom, a teenagers' lounge, and an auditorium. The health station eventually was replaced by the Altgeld Health Clinic. The public library still exists, but the nursery, teen lounge and auditorium are gone. The center of the development, called "Up top" by residents, contained a privately developed shopping center with a member-owned food co-op, doctor's offices, beauty and barbershops, and a tavern. The food co-op is now a grocery store, owned by non-resident Middle Eastern immigrants. The doctor's office, now called the Murray Clinic, is run by an immigrant doctor and several assistants. The beauty and barbershops still exist, but the tavern has been replaced with a liquor store.

Two new developments were built next to Altgeld Gardens. The first of these was Philip-Murray Homes, which has 500 units and was completed in the early 1950s. Then came Eden Green in 1968. This was the nation's first and largest black-owned and -operated development, with 800 units of townhouses and apartments (*Chicago Tribune* 02/21/82).

Economic Background: The economic outlook for this community, and a large part of the South Side, is bleak. Starting with the decline of the post-war industrial boom and the closing of the stockyards, steel mills, factories and other South Side industries the economic base for this community collapsed. The shrinking industrial base and subsequent loss of jobs over the last few decades have had a dramatic effect on these neighborhoods. Altgeld Gardens was once considered a model community for working class African American families;

instead it has become, in large part, a devastated community of the unemployed and underemployed dependent on public assistance. It ranks second among Chicago's seventy-seven community areas for its rate of infant mortality, thirteenth for its rate of births to mothers under twenty years of age, fifteenth for its rate of gonorrhea, eighth for its rate of chlamydia, and third for its rate of domestic violence against women eighteen and older (Community Area Health Inventory: CDPH Epidemiology Program Report 1996–1998, Vol. II: Rankings).

East Humboldt Park (EHP)

The community areas of West Town, Humboldt Park, and Logan Square (collectively referred to here as East Humboldt Park EHP) have some of the highest concentrations of individuals of Hispanic origin in Chicago: "The first wave of Puerto Rican immigration started in 1946, when Puerto Rico negotiated a labor contract to send five hundred persons here to work as laborers and domestics" (*Chicago Sun Times* 06/12/77). The second wave began about 1960, and in six years the number of Puerto Ricans increased from about 10,000 to 40,000 (*Chicago Sun Times* 06/14/66). These neighborhoods have experienced overall population decline during the past several decades with the largest occurring among white residents. Hispanic populations however have held steady, and in some cases increased. According to the 2000 census, EHP has a total combined population of 235,986 residents of which approximately 54% are Hispanic, 25% white, and 19% African American.

West Town, Humboldt Park, and Logan Square all border Humboldt Park, one of Chicago's oldest and largest parks and a location of significant drug activity and high-risk sexual behavior. Most of the housing stock in these communities was built in the early 1900s. Many sturdy brick structures with Victorian features were subdivided into smaller units to accommodate the demand for housing among Hispanic immigrants. The result in many cases was substandard, expensive housing, often neglected by absentee landlords. West Town, which borders a much more prosperous community of the Near North Side to the east, has experienced significant pressure from gentrification over the past fifteen years. From 1986 to 1991, home prices in West Town increased 20% a year (*Chicago Sun Times* 11/15/91). The shortage of affordable housing in the area coupled with the increased demand has forced many low- and moderate-income residents to move. The majority of EHP's residents are working class Hispanics, with some persons of Mexican descent. Among Chicago's seventy-seven community areas West Town, Humboldt Park, and Logan Square ranked sixteenth, nineteenth, and twenty-fourth, respectively, for the lowest average median income. They ranked seventeenth, sixteenth, and twenty-fourth, respectively, for areas with the highest percentage of residents living below poverty level (Community Area Health Inventory: CDPH Epidemiology Program Report 1996–1998, Vol. II: Rankings).

Additionally, EHP has a high concentration of injection drug users (IDUs). Heroin is the most prevalent injected drug, but the use of cocaine and other drugs is also common. HIV infection struck IDUs in the area early and hard. This was most likely due to contacts with HIV-positive drug injectors in or from Puerto Rico and New York City, where infection levels often exceeded 50% among IDUs. The high concentration of IDUs in EHP almost certainly accelerated the transmission of HIV once it entered these networks. In a 1988 study conducted by the University of Illinois at Chicago, almost 35% of IDUs in the EHP area were HIV positive. High mortality among IDUs infected early in the epidemic and a reduction in risky behaviors by current IDUs have reduced the rate of new HIV infections in these neighborhoods (Wiebel, Jimenez, Johnson et al. 1996; Ouellet, Jovanovic, Lampinen, et al. 1996). Humboldt Park ranks 14th in its percent of births to mothers under twenty years of age and 18th in its rate of infant mortality. It ranks sixteenth, twenty-second, and seventeenth respectively for its rates of syphilis, gonorrhea, and chlamydia (Community Area Health Inventory: CDPH Epidemiology Program Report 1996–1998, Vol. II: Rankings).

Far West Side

The RARE team's Far West Side assessment centered on Cicero Avenue between Roosevelt Road and North Avenue. The neighborhoods in this area are Austin, West Garfield Park and the western section of Humboldt Park. Once almost exclusively white neighborhoods, Austin and West Garfield Park experienced dramatic shifts in population in the last fifty years. Prior to 1960, Austin's population was almost exclusively white but by 1970 African Americans constituted one-third of residents. A major population shift took place that decade and by 1980 nearly three-quarters of the residents were black. West Garfield Park experienced an equally dramatic shift in population between 1950 and 1970. According to the 2000 Census, the community areas of Austin and West Garfield Park currently have populations that are 90% and 98% African American respectively.

Cicero Avenue is a mixed commercial and residential route that runs along a north/south axis on Chicago's far west side. It is bordered by Austin on the west, West Garfield Park on the southeast, and Humboldt Park on the northeast. The research team concentrated on a three-mile section that runs north from Roosevelt Road to North Avenue. This area contains many of the West Side's open-air drug markets, which are gang controlled and operate around the clock. While injection drug use has been common in this area, the concentration of IDUs appears not to be as great as in East Humboldt Park. Instead, the area's drug users are likely to smoke crack cocaine and 'snort' heroin.

During the white flight of the 1960s and 1970 Austin experienced a serious loss of industry as white businessmen left the neighborhood taking their businesses and jobs with them. As a result, Austin experienced economic downturns in the early 1970s and again in the early 1980s that the community is still trying to overcome. Although median household income in Austin is approximately $25,000 dollars (ranking it twenty-ninth among community areas), this obscures the disparity in income between Austin's less well-to-do southern residents and its much better-off northern residents. For example, in 1979 thirty-one percent of Austin's residents received public assistance and eighty-three percent of that went to south Austin (The Reader, 07/01/88). In 1998 the median household income for West Garfield Park was $15,102, placing it fourteenth among Chicago's community areas. Humboldt Park ranks nineteenth in income with a median of $20,038. Austin, Humboldt Park and West Garfield Park rank sixteenth, fifteenth and ninth respectively for their percentages of residents receiving public aid (Community Area Health Inventory: CDPH Epidemiology Program Report 1996–1998, Vol. II: Rankings).

Of Chicago's seventy-seven community areas, these three West Side areas together rank in the top one-quarter for their 1996–1998 rates of AIDS cases and mortality due to HIV infection. In addition, Austin and West Garfield Park rank nineteenth, and twelfth, respectively, for their rates of infant mortality, and fifteenth and thirteenth for their rates of births to mothers under twenty years of age. West Garfield Park ranks first for its homicide rate while Austin ranks thirteenth. The two rank eleventh and twelfth, respectively, for their rate of domestic violence against women eighteen and older. STD rates in these two communities are alarming. Austin and West Garfield Park rank sixth and first, respectively, for their syphilis rates, thirteenth and sixth for their gonorrhea rates, and fourth and seventh for their chlamydia rates (Community Area Health Inventory: CDPH Epidemiology Program Report 1996–1998, Vol. II: Rankings).

Findings

Injection Drug Use

Our teams observed the following among injection drug users in all four areas of study:

> Finding 1: Age trends in injection drug use differ by race/ethnicity and community area.
> Finding 2: Conditions exist for widespread mixing of different population groups.

For example, in Altgeld Gardens most of the IDUs tend to be long-time injectors over thirty years old. The number of young African Americans who inject drugs appears to be low, but difficult to estimate. Recent research suggests that injection drug use is highly stigmatized among young African Americans. Those who engage in this practice are particularly secretive. The most popular drugs for injection are heroin and a mix of heroin and cocaine (speedballs). Some whites, mostly over thirty years old, were seen purchasing drugs in Altgeld Gardens. Local residents told us it was not uncommon to see buyers driving vehicles with out-of-state license plates.

While whites tend to leave the Gardens as soon as they have purchased their drugs, residents told us that some use the apartments of resident IDUs to inject their drugs. Given that injection paraphernalia may be shared in these circumstances, it is likely that HIV, hepatitis and other pathogens are transmitted between these otherwise separate populations. Sex for money or drugs is likely to provide another means for spreading HIV from the Gardens to Chicago's Southeast Side, the southern suburbs and Northwest Indiana.

In East Humboldt Park, IDUs of all ages are easily found. White IDUs of all ages are also in the area and the number of those under thirty years old appears to be increasing. A small number of African American IDUs interact with these networks as well. Heroin is the drug most often used, although poly-drug use is common. Middle-aged Latino and white IDUs residing in this area commonly use drugs together. Further mixing between groups of IDUs may occur when East Humboldt Park IDUs travel to open-air drug markets in adjoining African American neighborhoods to purchase relatively high-quality heroin and cocaine at attractive prices. Drug users often prefer to use their drugs soon after purchase, so places exist to serve this need. It is likely that some EHP IDUs inject with African Americans in areas around the drug markets.

On the Far West Side, IDUs who reside in these largely African American neighborhoods tend to be long-time injectors over thirty years old, as well. According to a recent Drug Enforcement Agency estimate, this area contains over two hundred open-air drug markets specializing in heroin, crack cocaine and marijuana. These markets attract users from across metropolitan Chicago. Customers include African Americans from other areas of Chicago, Hispanics from adjoining neighborhoods and large numbers of whites. Observations by the RARE team, discussions with outreach workers serving this area and data from studies in this area indicate the majority of these whites are under thirty years old and use heroin, most intranasally. They come from areas on the Northwest Side including those neighborhoods populated by immigrants from Eastern Europe, gentrified areas on the near Northwest Side and suburban neighborhoods.

What are Their Injection Risk Practices?

Among IDUs, needle sharing represents the greatest risk for transmitting HIV. While this practice may never be eliminated, both the self-reports of persons interviewed by the RARE team and recent survey research conducted by investigators from the University of Illinois at Chicago (UIC) indicate that steep declines in needle sharing have occurred in some areas of Chicago over the past decade.

Finding 3: The more an area or population has access to needle exchange, street outreach and similar HIV-prevention programs, the less likely IDUs share needles.

Virtually every IDU contacted reported sharing syringes when s/he does not have access to a clean one. Two situations appear to account for this behavior. First, in an isolated, highly communal setting like the Gardens, the obligation IDUs feel to help one another is particularly intense. So IDUs share syringes with others who are without either their own drugs or syringe. Assistance implies reciprocation in the future. Social reciprocity makes it more likely that in the future the person providing the syringe will be helped when he or she is in need. Second, everyone contacted reported that there was no needle exchange program in the Gardens, and several expressed no knowledge of what a needle exchange program is. Some people reported buying needles from diabetics or other heroin users, sources that cannot be relied upon to always sell new unused needles. We were told of an underground needle exchange provider who does not charge money for needles. But this service appears to be sporadic and the demand for clean injection equipment clearly outweighs its availability.

In contrast, interviews done in East Humboldt Park indicate that needle sharing is uncommon among IDUs in this area. Those who share needles do so infrequently and with only one partner with whom they have a relationship, such as a friend or spouse. Needle sharing between strangers is rare. The relatively low level of needle sharing found here probably is linked to the extensive and longstanding presence of HIV-prevention services in this area. A variety of service providers target IDUs and two needle exchange programs provide extensive access to clean injection equipment, including during evening hours. Indigenous street outreach workers have promoted HIV-risk reduction here since at least 1986, and a methadone treatment program is available locally. All IDUs interviewed by the team were familiar with the area's needle exchange programs and most were aware of the presence of street outreach workers.

On the Far West Side, the potential for needle sharing among the middle-aged African American IDUs appears low. Occasional needle sharing was reported during the team's interviews, but most IDUs expressed an intent and ability not to share needles. As in Humboldt Park, two needle exchange programs make clean needles available five days a week. However, the area served by these programs is relatively large, thus IDUs have to travel farther than those in East Humboldt Park to reach a site. Most IDUs were aware of the needle exchange programs, though the proportion was lower than in Humboldt Park. Recent research with young white IDUs who frequent the West Side to buy and use drugs indicate that they remain at high risk for sharing needles. First, they appear not to have been introduced to drug injection by older IDUs, the group most likely to practice—and perhaps teach—safer injection. Second, until recently, young white IDUs were woefully ignorant of the availability of HIV prevention services such as needle exchange. However, many remain at risk even when they use services such as needle exchange because they live with their parents and are afraid to store clean needles at home.

According to a local service provider, until recently street outreach workers regularly accessed 'shooting galleries' on the West Side and linked them to the needle exchange programs. Shooting galleries are places IDUs utilize for the purpose of injecting drugs. A typical shooting gallery is operated by an IDU and located in his or her apartment, for which the price of admission is a 'taste' of one's drugs. Galleries often provide injection equipment and some include a 'house doctor' who is proficient at injecting IDUs who are unable to inject themselves or unable to find a usable vein. Shooting galleries are prime locations for HIV transmission, because the same injection equipment may be rented or loaned to multiple IDUs from a variety of areas around the neighborhood or city. Street outreach workers have worked for years to identify shooting galleries and convince their operators to make safer injection practices the norm in their galleries. In the past, outreach workers made sure galleries had locked 'sharps' containers to dispose of their patron's needles immediately after they were used. Full containers were returned to the needle exchange program for safe disposal. Several providers interviewed for this report indicated that funding restrictions for needle exchange programs make it difficult to continue this work on a regular basis.

What Are the Settings for Risk?

> Finding 4: The public housing site's isolation, lack of access to legal employment, and lack of services contribute to drug use and HIV risk.
>
> Finding 5: Gentrification in some areas is changing how drugs are used, in ways that both increase and decrease the risk for HIV transmission.

Altgeld Gardens is one of the most socio-economically devastated communities in Chicago. Among Chicago's seventy-seven community areas, the area in which the Gardens is located ranked fifth in the 1990 Census for the proportion of children living in families whose annual income fell below the poverty level (76%) and seventh for the proportion of residents receiving Public Aid (62%). In 1990, only 56% of persons aged twenty-five and older had graduated from high school, and the community area's unemployment rate ranked second in the city. Compounding these problems, the Gardens are geographically isolated, with limited public transportation, on the city's south side. Residents repeatedly conveyed a sense of separation from the worlds of work and commerce in Chicago. In the face of such tremendous problems, residents still reported a scarcity of social programs designed to offset the multidimensional social and psychological consequences of sustained poverty. One focus group participant offered her reflections on why so many young men in the Gardens traffic in drugs:

> A lot of people out here can work on cars and stuff, but look how far you have to go to get to be a certified mechanic . . . Look at what you got to go through to be a certified plumber. A lot of guys would probably be interested in carpentry school and stuff. But then they never been shown how they could go about doing it. For a lot of them it's their egos. Cause a lot of them just want the spotlight. If you can't get no-where, you sell drugs. If you don't know but one way of life, you going to do only what you know.

Not surprisingly, reports from several residents suggest that dope houses (or drug use "spots") exist throughout the Gardens. The team witnessed drug sales taking place at various locations and times on virtually every trip to the Gardens. As one drives through the neighborhood, young men selling drugs are a common sight as they talk on cell phones and connect with buyers who arrive in cars and on foot. One heroin injector said, "Ain't nothing out here. Ain't nothing but the dope houses . . . Where you go you ain't seeing nothing but dope cause there ain't nothing to do but come up here, drink and get high, and then go back home, probably eat, come back up and try it again."

East Humboldt Park is experiencing the same gentrification pressures that began pushing IDUs out of West Town in the 1980s. Observations by the RARE team and reports of IDUs they interviewed indicated that one of the effects of this change is that illicit drug-related activities have become more clandestine and mobile. Rather than there being sustained "pockets of risk," today persons selling and using drugs regularly move in response to pressure from police and citizens, and open-air drug dealing has increasingly given way to transactions arranged through beepers and telephones. In the park itself, landscaping changes eliminated a large area of foliage used by hundreds of IDUs for cover while injecting drugs. During the period of observation, there was little drug dealing in the park, although this may change as winter gives way to warmer weather.

Humboldt Park used to contain numerous shooting galleries, but the team found that increased police pressure and fewer abandoned buildings—both linked to gentrification—have led to a notable decline in the number of these informal drug-use sites. A respected street outreach worker noted that it is more difficult now to get IDUs to reveal the locations of shooting galleries for fear that word will get around and that the police will take action.

Sexual HIV Risk

What are the risk practices?

> Finding 6: Condom use is practiced most often between casual partners and least often between primary partners.
> Finding 7: In the sex trade, condom use is practiced most often by those who sell sex for money and least often by those who trade sex for drugs.

> Finding 8: Many sexworkers interviewed for this report stated that police have been citing simple condom possession as probable cause for a prostitution arrest.

There is also the perception among many sexworkers that repeated arrests for prostitution can result in a felony charge. Sexworkers seeking to avoid arrest and prosecution may tend not to carry and utilize condoms when selling sex on the street. In addition, they are likely to trade sex for drugs in drug houses where they have least control over clients.

In Altgeld Gardens, assessments of unprotected sex rely mainly on self-reports, but young children can serve as a marker (marker?) for unprotected sex. The field assessment team noted that in the Gardens there are many children of teen mothers. When asked if there is a lot of unsafe sex in the Gardens, one female participant in a focus group stated the following:

> Everywhere you look its a stroll. Winter's coming now; wait till the summer and see all the strollers. All these young girls having babies. That's all they do is have babies. More babies, more babies, more babies, every time I look around. Girls twelve and thirteen years old are having babies in the seventh and eighth grades. They got no alternatives, so what they going to do? Ain't no place for them to go. All they got to do is walk around and have sex, what else?

According to several residents interviewed by the team, many women in their twenties and older, trade sex for drugs. In particular, young women provide sex to drug dealers in return for drugs. According to one young woman who uses drugs, "The sex is all about crack. There is no more selling sex for money. It is now a trade for crack." Preventing AIDS is far from anyone's mind.

In East Humboldt Park, data suggest that the use of condoms is increasingly accepted for sex between casual partners, but is far less common for sex between primary partners. Among the area's female sexworkers, condom use is well accepted, but they reported two problems. First, free condoms are not always available for several reasons. The sex worker may not have been around when the outreach workers who serve these areas were present. Outreach typically takes place during the day, while sex work is done at night and in the early morning. HIV-prevention funding increasingly emphasizes office rather than street-based services. Even when sexworkers have a supply of condoms, they may use them faster than expected or have to throw them away before being approached by police. Several sexworkers reported some reluctance about carrying condoms because police officers use condoms as evidence that the women were currently engaged in prostitution.

A second barrier to condom use reported by sexworkers is resistance by male customers. Some men apply pressure to forego condom use, typically by threatening to take their business elsewhere or by offering more money. Since sexworkers experience considerable competition for customers and most are poor and addicted to crack cocaine or heroin, they find it difficult to refuse men who do not want to use condoms. Sexworkers also reported considerable concern that a new law will allow the State to charge them with a felony for engaging in prostitution after repeated arrests. Given that most of these women regularly use heroin or crack cocaine, it seems plausible that more will move away from soliciting sex on the street and instead trade sex directly for drugs in venues such as crack houses where HIV infection is almost guaranteed.

Finding 9: Unprotected sex involving sexworkers provides a path for infection transmission between residents of the city and suburbs.

At all three sites, sexworkers are primarily women in their 20s and 30s who reflect the racial/ethnic composition of their respective area. Most regularly use heroin and/or crack cocaine. Trans-gendered (male-to-female) sexworkers are present in both East Humboldt Park and the Far West Side. Customers of sexworkers in both East Humboldt Park and the Far West Side are a mix of two groups. One group is composed of local men who typically approach the women on foot or in cars or patronize them in drug houses. This group is comprised of those most likely to offer drugs rather than money for sex, and to have sex in low-rent hotels, abandoned buildings or drug houses. Another group is composed of men from other areas of the city, the suburbs and elsewhere. These men typically pay money for sex, have sex in their automobiles, and are more likely to offer more money not to use condoms.

HIV Prevention Services

Finding 10: Most IDUs have been counseled and tested for HIV. However, many have not gotten results recently and few are being tested as often as their risk practices warrant.

At all sites except Altgeld Gardens nearly everyone reported having been counseled and tested for HIV. However, most people the teams spoke with were not getting tested every six months even though they continued to engage in behaviors that placed them at risk for HIV infection, and even fewer returned for their test results.

Finding 11: The provision of HIV prevention services at the various sites is uneven and no site appeared to have adequate intervention programming at night.
Finding 12: Ancillary services that compliment HIV prevention are often absent or not clearly visible to high-risk populations.
Finding 13: Residents of isolated, insular communities like Altgeld Gardens often avoid local-based services because they fear that confidentiality will be breached.

In Altgeld Gardens, one agency regularly offered HIV-prevention programming using indigenous outreach workers who were familiar with local drug injection and sexwork scenes. Most IDUs we interviewed recognized this agency's red van and knew of their services. But the agency was not able to sustain funding or to maintain its apartment service center which provided a variety of other HIV-prevention services. The local Altgeld Health Clinic offers free condoms that are placed in a small bowl in their office, and they began an HIV counseling and testing program in December 2000. However, most of the residents we spoke with were not aware of these services. Residents cited no other HIV-prevention services other than occasional HIV testing by outside groups that they perceived as 'just coming and going.'

All IDUs the team spoke with reported that they would use prevention programs if they were available. One woman told us, "Okay, so if I'm using and you tell me that these needles going to kill me, well hell I ain't got none (clean needles). So maybe if you had some kind of program, I can get some." Several people commented that the Local Advisory Council has been opposed for some time to the idea of a needle exchange program in the Gardens. The Council's role is to serve as a voice of the community and, in particular, as a liaison between residents and the Chicago Housing Authority and the city.

Not only are there virtually no HIV-prevention services, there are no drug addiction treatment programs or help centers in the Gardens either. Many study participants expressed a lack of knowledge about outside services. One man's comment was typical: "I don't know of any programs in or even outside of the Gardens that people go to get help except the rehab center. I've heard people speak about it, but don't know where it is." A woman who injects drugs described more graphically the lack of substance abuse treatment services in the following conversation:

> Q: What about services for people who use drugs, injection drug users? Are there any places they can go for rehabilitation inside this community?
> Respondent: Is she for real? You get no damn rehabilitation out here.
> Q: So we already know that there's not a needle exchange program and there is not a methadone program. And so, say for instance if a person wanted to go into rehab, what would be the procedure? How would they do it?
> Respondent: Overdose. Let the hospital send you somewhere. You can't go in there and say 'I'm on my last leg. I'm trying to do something.' The Department of Human Services is gone. The people up here don't know shit. Don't nobody know what to tell you. We will pray for you.' You can't go nowhere and just be sent somewhere. Somebody say, 'Let me look in the book and see who got a bed for you.' You get high till you OD. Ambulance take you

> somewhere, Roseland Hospital. If they don't kill you, then you go and get you some help.

In addition to an absence of HIV and drug-related services, residents reported a lack of other social services for adults and children, as well as a lack of programs to help residents gain employment. The team met one young college graduate who said he had had no idea of how to get a job after graduating and, instead, returned to the Gardens where he became immersed in drug trafficking and use. The isolation of the Gardens from the city clearly makes it even more difficult—both logistically and psychologically—for residents to seek outside services or employment. The Gardens present a serious dilemma for service planners. On the one hand, residents feel isolated and hesitate to leave the Gardens for services. On the other hand, residents worry that problems they share with any service provider located in the Gardens will become known to other residents. This fear is particularly great when local service providers employ persons who reside within the tight-knit community of the Gardens.

In contrast, East Humboldt Park has a number of service providers that address HIV prevention, substance abuse and other medical and social needs. The area's needle exchange programs were known by all IDUs with whom the team spoke and the majority was aware of street outreach. Substance abusers who did not inject drugs were less aware of outreach programs and all groups either had less than optimal awareness of other programs or were confusion about where, when and how to obtain other services.

On the Far West Side, there are also several service providers that provide programs addressing HIV prevention, substance abuse and/or other medical and social needs. Again, the needle exchange programs are widely known, but there is less awareness of other programs. Ignorance or confusion about HIV prevention and related service programs seemed greatest among high-risk non-IDUs such as crack smokers, and young sexworkers who were active late at night.

Recommendations

> Recommendation 1: In or near Altgeld Gardens, establish a needle exchange program accompanied by case management and consistent street outreach that promotes HIV-risk reduction.

To ensure credibility and confidentiality, the case managers should be people familiar with injection drug use but not residents of the Gardens. Consideration should be given to using one of the many empty units at The Gardens as a base for case management and street outreach.

> Recommendation 2: At the least, IDUs and other substance abusers need someone based in or near the Gardens who can guide them to existing services.

At Altgeld Gardens, the sense of isolation and hopelessness among residents is striking, even when compared to other low-income communities. To ensure confidentiality, such a person should not be a resident. The needs of those addicted to drugs might best be served by a treatment center that has a referral site in the Gardens and a clinic outside the Gardens. Beyond these steps, a wide range of services are needed for both children and adults. Service planning at the Gardens needs to be particularly sensitive to the reluctance of residents to leave the community for services, while also fearing that confidentiality will be breached if they seek help locally.

> Recommendation 3: Service providers in East Humboldt Park and on the Far West Side should work together not only to better link their services, but also to make the linkages more visible to persons at high risk for contracting or transmitting HIV.

For example, services providers should consider producing a pamphlet that, as simply as possible, directs members of high-risk populations to a range of existing services in the community.

> Recommendation 4: Conduct street outreach at night that targets sexworkers and young substance abusers.

Agencies indicate that this may require additional funds to do on a consistent basis. The main goals of such outreach would be to provide HIV-prevention materials at a time when they may be otherwise unavailable and to bring persons at high risk for contracting or transmitting HIV into other existing HIV-prevention services.

> Recommendation 5: CDPH should work with the Chicago Police Department to educate its police force on the strong connections between unprotected sex and the spread of HIV and other STDs.

As such, this dialogue should address the problems with reported police practices that correlate condom possession with sex work, and therefore set up barriers to the use of condoms by sex workers.

> Recommendation 6: Increase the availability of harm reduction supplies, including condoms and sterile syringes.

This may be done through outreach programs, needle exchange programs and by making syringes legally available without prescription. Regarding the latter strategy, Illinois is now one of only five states that require a prescription to purchase sterile syringes.

Afterward

The final report and recommendations for Chicago's RARE project were submitted to the Office of Mayor Richard M. Daley on Wednesday, September 3, 2001, and again on October 3, 2001. The findings were made available to the public on November 15, 2001. While there was no direct response from the Mayor's office regarding the report, the STD/HIV/AIDS Division of the Department of Health did incorporate the findings from the report into the planning processes of both the HIV/AIDS Planning Group and the Title I services planning. CDPH staff formally presented the findings to each of the committees and members of each of these committees were provided with copies of the report and its findings. Additionally, a copy of the report was provided to each of Chicago's city council members. Finally, the AIDS Foundation of Chicago used information contained in the report during its campaign to gain increased funds for the Department of Health, Division of STD/HIV/AIDS for HIV/AIDS prevention and care programs. While the report cannot be credited for the $600,000 in increased FY04 funds received by the Department of Health as a result of this campaign, its findings did highlight the need for increased HIV/AIDS-prevention and care services in Chicago, particularly targeting IDU, MSM and sexworker populations.

References

Bowley, Jr., Devereux (1978) *The Poorhouse: Subsidized Housing in Chicago 1895–1976*. Carbondale, Illinois: Southern Illinois University Press.

Ouellet, L.J., Thorpe, L.E., Huo, D., et al. (2000) "Prevalence and Incidence of HIV among Out-of-Treatment Injecting Drug Users, Chicago 1994–1996." *J. Acquir Immune Defic Syndr*. 25: 443–450.

Shore, Debra (1995) "The House that Gautreax Built" in University of Chicago Magazine, 87 (3): February.

Wiebel, W.W., Jimenez A.D., Johnson, W.A., et al. (1996) "Risk behavior and HIV Seroincidence among Out-of-Treatment Injection Drug Users: a Four Year Prospective Study." *J Acquir Immune Defic Syndr*. 12: 282–289.

Chapter 5

Confined Youth Trying to Make it Real, Despite the Odds: RARE in Baltimore

Ernest Quimby

Baltimore's Political Economy

It is not enough, perhaps even incorrect and certainly ineffective, to simply say that particular people and communities are at high risk for HIV/AIDS. The epidemic exists within a system of ongoing structured community-destabilization and it is undermining the ability of those threatened by the disease to exercise cultural values and norms that ensure their survival. The unrelenting onslaught of HIV/AIDS has accelerated alienation of people at the bottom of Baltimore's political economy. Globalization, political dismissal, racial subordination, social stigma and bureaucratic unresponsiveness are ongoing. Meanwhile, the public health crises of inner-city African Americans are much less important than maintaining a baseball or football stadium.

Statistical profiles of Baltimore indicate that its working class residents are faced with the immense burdens of economic want and government neglect and chronic social disruption, all of which compete with HIV/AIDS as public issues. These are evident when the following are considered: education, literacy, employment, poverty and low-income workers, poverty and children, recipients of welfare and Temporary Assistance for Needy Families (TANF), homelessness, and juvenile and criminal justice.

Education

In 2002, the percentage of out-of-school and out-of-work youth in the Baltimore metropolitan area was 13.5% of all youth sixteen to nineteen years old (35,900) when compared to Maryland's average of 12.8% (72,492). The percentage of Baltimore City youth, sixteen to nineteen years old, who were not in school and not working (18%), was twice that of youth in the Baltimore metropolitan area (9.8%) and Maryland (8.5%) at the time of the 2000 Census (Census, 2000; AYPF, 1997).

Literacy

In 1998, 38% of Baltimore's adults functioned between first and fourth grade reading levels. They were presumably unable to perform basic and important functions which are dependent on literacy and writing skills. That is, they are unable to determine their eligibility from a table of employee benefits, identify and write information on a Social Security card application or calculate total purchase costs from an order form.

Employment

Between 1990 and 2000, the proportion of the people in Baltimore City considered "not in the labor force" increased 4% from 39% to 43%. Such persons stopped looking for work because they retired, were discouraged or decided to remain in school (Census 2000). In 2002, large-scale layoffs in the Baltimore region almost doubled (4,726) those during the same period in the preceding year (2,850).

Poverty and Low-Income Workers

Approximately 135,630 people in Baltimore City live in poverty, including 52, 976 children under eighteen years old and 82,654 adults. In 1999, almost half (47%) of all Baltimore City families earned less than $35,000 compared to 25% of Maryland families. Between 1990 and 2000, Baltimore City median family "money" income increased 26% from $28,217 in 1990 to $35,438 in 2000. However, this was not a real increase. The Consumer Price Index estimated that the cost of living rose by 27.5% during the same time period. For the State of Maryland, median family income increased by 37% from $45,289 in 1990 to $61,876 in 2000. Census 2000 data indicate that 18.80% of families in Baltimore live below poverty, contrasted with 6.1% of families in Maryland. A higher number and concentration of low-skill jobs were outside Baltimore City than in the State of Maryland in 2000. Sixty-six percent (257,495 jobs) of employment in Baltimore City is classified as low-skill, compared to 69% to 72% in surrounding suburban counties (JOTF, 1999; Census 2000).

Poverty and Recipients of Welfare

In Baltimore City, in 2000, 31% of children lived at 100% of poverty. An additional 57% lived at 200% of poverty (Census 2000). The largest recipient of Temporary Assistance for Needy Families (TANF) Block Grant in Maryland is Baltimore City. As of September 2000 in Baltimore City, there were 13,813 "Paid TANF Cases with Adult" and 3,179 "Long-Term Cases with Adult." Twenty-three percent of all cases were long-term. As of September 2000, Maryland cases received TANF for at least thirty-six of the last forty-five months. Reductions in Baltimore City's cash assistance welfare caseloads significantly lagged behind suburban decreases over the last five years. Thus, 83% of area recipients are in Baltimore City. The Department of Human Resources indicates that 42.2% of households in Baltimore City received food stamps in 1999 (AYPF, 1997). Estimates of the homeless population in Baltimore City range between 2,400 and 3,000 people. Approximately 1,300 to 1,600 of Baltimore's homeless population have been incarcerated at some time.

Criminal and Juvenile Justice

During 2002, some 8,695 inmates were released by the State of Maryland to Baltimore City and scheduled for expiration, parole or mandatory supervision. They included 8,122 males and 573 females (PSCS, 2002). Arrest rates per 10,000 youth, ages 10–17, were between 100 and 120 in Baltimore City, in 1999, compared to 60 per 10,000 youth in the state of Maryland. In 1999, an estimated 6,271 petitioned delinquency court case counts formally reached court in Baltimore City. An additional 2,655 were non-petitioned delinquency court cases that did not have formal court proceedings (NCJJ, 1999).

Social and economic indicators and "snapshots" of Baltimore City and one of RARE's research sites reveal contexts which contribute to public health problems. These statistics are presented in tables 1 and 2. Again, HIV/AIDS exists within this set of economic, social, political and cultural environments that constrain responses of Baltimore's residents and policy officials.

Table 5.1: Glimpses of Baltimore City and Greenmount Community

	Baltimore City	Greenmount
Population (% African American)	651,154 (64%)	99 (99%)
Percent Living in Poverty	23%	23%
Median Household Income	$30,078	$23,958
Median Rent (% of median HH income)	$498 (20%)	$329 (16%)
Percent of Owner Occupied Housing Units	43%	30%
Percent of Families Headed by Single Mothers with Juvenile Children	52%	71%
Percent of Working-age Residents Relying on Public Transportation	20%	41%

Source: Smith and Steele, 2003

HIV/AIDS Epidemiological Overview

Throughout the U.S., African Americans disproportionately experience preventable and treatable diseases. These health disparities include cancer, cardiovascular diseases, stokes and HIV/AIDS, among other diseases (HHS 2000; IOM 2002; CDC 1998, 1999). In 1998, the Congressional Black Caucus requested the U.S. Department of Health and Human Services to declare HIV/AIDS a public health emergency in African American communities.

HIV/AIDS statistics by jurisdiction, gender and race for the Baltimore region remain grim. According to a Centers for Disease Control and Prevention (CDC) HIV/AIDS Surveillance Report, as of December 2000, the national annual AIDS incidence (new) rate was 14.7 cases per 100,000 population. Maryland's rate of 27.7 cases per 100,000 was the fifth highest of any state. The Baltimore metropolitan area rate (38.1 cases per 100,000) was the eighth highest of all metropolitan areas in the United States.

Data from Maryland Department of Health and Mental Hygiene, as of June 30, 2001, also revealed a serious situation. The Baltimore metropolitan area accounted for 66.6% (7,914) of cumulative AIDS deaths in Maryland. Baltimore

City accounted for nearly 52% of Maryland's reported HIV/AIDS cases. A closer statistical look at Baltimore City indicated a disturbing overview. An epidemic of staggering consequences stalked the city, attacked certain groups and threatened to ravage their communities. Baltimore is to this day under siege. A statistical portrait is provided below.

Table 5.2: HIV/AIDS in Baltimore City (June 30, 2001)

Measure	Number	Percent
Total HIV/AIDS Cases	11,512	51.9% of Maryland
Cumulative AIDS Deaths	6,437	54.2% of Maryland
Male HIV/AIDS Cases	7,271	63.3% of Baltimore City
Female HIV/AIDS Cases	4,212	36.7% of Baltimore City
African American AIDS Cases	9,335	88.9% of Baltimore City
White HIV/AIDS Cases	1,081	10.1% of Baltimore City
Hispanic HIV/AIDS Cases	49	0.5% of Baltimore City

Source: State of Maryland (2001). Dept. Health and Mental Hygiene.

In Baltimore City zip code 21217, there were nine hundred ninety total HIV/AIDS cases (8.6% of the city total) and six hundred forty-one cumulative AIDS deaths (10% Of the city total). An emergency response was needed to rapidly assess, respond to and evaluate HIV/AIDS programs in order to stem the epidemic in destabilized communities (HHS 1999; Trotter and Needle 1999). Baltimore's attempt is described in the following section.

Baltimore RARE Objectives

Baltimore RARE was a federal-local health initiative funded by the U.S. Department of Health and Human Services, Office of HIV/AIDS Policy (OHAP) and CDC, in response to a request for assistance from Baltimore City political and health officials (Needle et al. 2003). The project's objectives were to identify and describe types, places and times when behaviors engaged in by youth put them at extreme risk for contracting and spreading HIV/AIDS. The aim was to explain such activities in order to help Baltimore City Health Department

(BCHD) develop effective interventions. BCHD targeted youth 18–24 years old living in postal zones 21217 and 21218.

Process

The processes of initiation, engagement, implementation and evaluation were as follows: Baltimore's mayor requested federal financial and logistical assistance. The mayor and public health officials agreed on the roles and expectations of the local health department and federal officials. A research field team coordinator/ethnographer and a team liaison were then selected. Three teams of three members each were recruited. Training and planning were undertaken. Additional training was provided during the project. Field research data collection, reporting, analysis and assessment were conducted. Project data findings were synthesized into discrete thematic categories for refined analysis and subsequent continuous reporting to health officials. A final Field Research Report of research objectives, process, questions, methodology, findings, recommendations and conclusions was prepared. This document was presented for study, discussion, clarification and consideration for action steps.

Research Questions

A set of questions developed by the research team for focus groups and in-depth individual interviews was forwarded to BCHD's Institutional Review Board (IRB). After nearly two months, BCHD's IRB revised and approved the following questions to be probed during focus groups and interviews with community residents and service providers:

1. What is HIV/AIDS, and how does someone contract it?
2. Do youth, eighteen to twenty-four years old, consider HIV/AIDS to be a major problem in your neighborhood?
3. How concerned are teenagers in your neighborhood about getting HIV/AIDS?
4. What are teenagers saying or doing about their concerns?
5. How concerned do teenagers think parents/grandparents are about their children/grandchildren getting HIV/AIDS?
6. What are parents/grandparents saying or doing about their concerns?
7. What behaviors are putting youth, eighteen to twenty-four years old, at risk for getting HIV/AIDS?
8. When and where do these behaviors take place?
9. What types of HIV/AIDS services are in your neighborhood? Who uses them, and why?
10. Are these services considered worthwhile? Why or why not?

11. What types of HIV/AIDS-prevention services would you, or youth eighteen to twenty-four years old, most likely use?
12. Do people in your neighborhood think an HIV vaccine should be part of an HIV/AIDS-prevention program?
13. What types of HIV/AIDS-treatment services would you, or youth eighteen to twenty-four years old, most likely use?
14. How can the Baltimore City Health Department help reduce the spread of HIV/AIDS in your neighborhood?

Research Participants, Sites and Methods

Male and female African American youth, ages eighteen to twenty-four, who lived in the research sites were the principal targets. Data were also obtained from adult residents, business proprietors and community-based service providers.

Team members initially observed three zones (21215, 21217 and 21218) for a twenty-four-hour period. Observations were recorded every 15 to 45 minutes. When the location changed, each person documented the street and zip code area. Observation recording forms contained the observer's name, observation date, location of observation, summary notes, start and end times, and observer's comments. Further field investigations and mapping also took place. The broad postal sites were then narrowed down to specific blocks in Greenmount after observations of the entire area and increasingly narrow canvassing.

The field team conducted the following tasks: mapping, systematic observations, focus groups, in-depth formal interviewing, brief informal interviews, street intercepts, conversations, field notes, debriefing, data reporting, data analysis and street outreach. Prior to formal interviews and focus groups, the project's purpose, procedures, risks, benefits, voluntary nature and alternative to participation, and confidentiality safeguards were clearly described in an informed consent form approved by BCHD's Institutional Review Board. After the project's purpose and informed consent form were verbally explained and discussed, each participating focus group member or interviewee read and voluntarily signed the informed consent form. A separate form was used for focus groups and interviews. Participants were reimbursed $20.00. They were able to refuse to answer any question and could withdraw from the focus group or interview at any time.

Site team researchers prepared, presented and critically reviewed their maps, observations and reports with the overall team. They prepared field notes, interpreted findings and generated preliminary recommendations. Suggestions for improving the research were shared. Researchers also did limited HIV/AIDS street outreach as a way of engaging participants. The field team coordinator/ethnographer organized field work, conducted weekly de-briefing meetings, reviewed data collection methods, analyzed data, and served as a liaison between federal and local health officials.

Weekly meetings were held at BCHD and community sites. Team debriefings and training emphasized thoroughness of reporting, attentiveness to details and specificity focused on people, activities, times, reasons, places and consequences. Team members gave critical, yet supportive suggestions for improving the quality of data collection and reporting. Members were continuously cautioned and critiqued to provide descriptions and assessments that avoided judgmental or presumptuous reporting.

Description of Greenmount

Greenmount is a low-income, African American, inner-city neighborhood. Residents are suspicious of outsiders. The community is a tight-knit East Baltimore area. Some of it appears to be a war zone, perhaps more in attitude and behaviors, but also in certain physical respects.

The neighborhood can be dangerous after 10 p.m., because of drug dealing activities. In some areas, drug use is very heavy. Stumbling and nodding off, people look and act as if they are high or intoxicated, based on how they walk, talk and look. Police efforts have been initiated to reduce situations that may lead to crime and violence. Plainclothes officers will suddenly pull up to a spot, leap from their unmarked cars, and frisk everyone. One or two youth may be arrested. Sometimes officers pour alcohol from confiscated bottles. Between 11 p.m. and 7 a.m., police impose strict anti-loitering restrictions. A "Hands Across Baltimore" campaign has been launched, consisting of community-based organizations and city government.

However, such actions do not cramp the drug trade or curtail open-air drug markets. As police approach, an alert is sounded and teenagers scurry for cover. Drug "shops" open as soon as police cruisers are out of sight, even if dealers are arrested, handcuffed, placed on the ground for transport, and eventually hauled away. It takes longer for arresting officers to wait for another police car than for dealers to resume their trading places.

People sit on their stoops. Children play ball and ride in the streets. Adults go and come from bars, liquor stores and carry-outs. They visit friends and converse with neighbors. A favorite place to wait is at a fresh frozen fruit drink stand. A steamed crab truck also does a steady business. Money comes into the community, but leaves just as quickly. Certain pleasures such as drug use are immediate, but expensive when repeatedly sought. There are people who will deliver services to pleasure seekers for any price—this is a major source of income when there are no others.

Spotters are on most corners. For example, an African American male, seventeen to twenty years old, dressed in a black t-shirt, jeans and Timberland boots is one such person. Other youth, sixteen to twenty, wait for his directions. He is the one, "our boy," who runs the corner. Activity is happening or is about to happen. Males and females, youth and adults, individually, in pairs or groups of three or four, on foot and by car, begin to gradually approach the t-shirted youth—not all at once, but over a period of hours. A ritual unfolds. Brief words and quick negotiation take place. He is given money. Then he crosses the street, enters an alley, goes to the back of the second house from the corner, retrieves a small package, returns to the other side of the street, and hands it over to whoever gave him the money. His boys stroll up and down the block, glancing warily, casually, in whatever way that allows them to be good lookouts without drawing attention to themselves. This youth, brazenly dealing on the corner, is a leader. He also has opportunities to "fry" (have sex with) females who approach him because of his status.

Occasionally whites, generally young males and females (with black women and men) can also be spotted buying drugs. One or two white women sometimes are out tricking (engaging in prostitution). An African American woman stands on a corner drinking her "forty" (40 oz. beer bottle) in a brown paper bag. Other women and men sit on the steps of an abandoned store to cop drugs.

Findings

Our research detected significant major community issues in Greenmount that affect residents' ability to protect themselves from HIV by controlling their social structures and embracing HIV-preventive lifestyles. These dynamics are thematically described below.

Barriers to Reducing HIV/AIDS among Youth

Many youth, families, adults and peers have not embraced ownership or acknowledgement of HIV/AIDS. Various factors directly retard outreach, prevention and treatment. According to focus groups and interviews, obstacles faced by youth include: stigma, fear, suspicion, alienation, incorrect or outdated HIV/AIDS information, rumors, scarcity of readily available services, unwillingness to use existent services, minimal resources, lack of forums for receiving information and discussing attitudes, absence of community development, non-direction, lack of structured support, absence of formal leadership, lack of indigenous leadership, shortage of outlets, perceptions of morality, guilt, uncertainty of one's HIV status and an unwillingness to share one's HIV status with significant others.

Separate interviews, conversations and focus groups with youth and adults revealed a set of factors and patterns of circumstances and behaviors that promote the contraction and spread of HIV/AIDS, and retard treatment efforts. The indicators most often cited by residents were the following: 1) destabilizing drugs, 2) conflicting sexual pressures, 3) disturbing gender patterns, 4) minimal parental influence, 5) negative environmental influences, 6) depressing economic conditions, 7) inadequate services, and 8) competing attitudes and perceptions. They are described in subsequent sections.

1. Destabilizing Drugs

Drugs are sold day and night. In the early morning, sales are low. Morning drug dealing activity is noticeable as early as 7 a.m. Dealing increases in the afternoon. It intensifies after 8 p.m. By late evening, after 8 p.m., foot and vehicle traffic can be heavy. The drugs of choice by youth are marijuana, cocaine and heroin.

Youth, generally seventeen to twenty years old, although some are younger, are "into alcohol." Young males ride by on bikes carrying and sipping liquor from bottles in brown paper bags. Intense drug sales by youth, ages seventeen to twenty-five, can last until 2 a.m. On Greenmount and Lorraine Avenues, a group of six African American males run up to different cars, yelling various street names for cocaine and marijuana.

Neighborhood drug dealing is run by tightly organized youth. Hand signals are used to indicate one is selling drugs, e.g., advertising weed by placing one's thumb and index finger together as if smoking. Older dealers (19+) often have younger runners, wearing black and white bandannas, who serve as liaisons by running back and forth to attract and negotiate with customers. Sometimes, from late evening to early morning (8 p.m. to 2 a.m.), these young people are on the corner of Barclay and 20th, and share a pint of Hennessy bought by a male (twenty-one to twenty-three year old) who emerges from a car. Some females hold a small black purse over their shoulders, possibly to stash drugs. The youth may be waiting for potential buyers. Females appear to be just hanging. Their role may be to keep younger children in check, sit on steps or stand in certain spots and look out for the man. Groups of "hoppers" (adolescents and very young adults) seem to control neighborhoods. Some have cell phones. Many ride bikes. The drug dealing area is structured and administered by youth with definable areas: Barclay Boys sell cocaine and heroin. Lorraine Boys, "where the girls are," push coke and weed. The Greenmount crew merchandises everything. Weed is peddled by guys at 24th and Barclay and Cokesbury Streets.

Most street dealers are not independent entrepreneurs even if they appear to be working alone. They hustle for someone else. About 7 p.m., on the corner of Greenmount and Worsley, a young male sells a bag of ready rock (crack) to two females, one black and the other white. Other females cop from him. Then two black males, twenty-six to twenty-eight years old, pull up and get out from a Lexus. They talk to the dealer for a few minutes and get money from him. Many people he serves come from outside the area.

Main drug selling and using sites are alleys, houses, apartment buildings, abandoned dwellings, cars, SUVs, Jeeps and street corners. Many abandoned buildings are used as shooting galleries. Stores are generally places for drug sales, but not drug use. Much drug activity takes place in a little alley at Worsley and Greenmount from 6 a.m. to 3 p.m. the following day.

Sometimes, the drug business can be assertive. Street youth dealers establish rights and rites of dominance. They may abuse their customers. Youth will boldly tout drugs to motorists and pedestrians. Ten male youth (ages eighteen to twenty-one) lean on parked cars. They start chasing and flagging down cars, screaming the colors of their bags of weed, cocaine and ready rock. As people ride down the street, young dealers hang on their car doors, attempting to get a sale.

The drug trade is relentless and omnipresent. Loch Raven and Cokesbury Street is a major site of marijuana, beer and other alcohol use by youth. Greenmount Avenue Park at 24th Street is known for its marijuana sales. Major drug deals occur around Greenmount and 21st, Barclay and 21st, Lorraine and Barclay, and Cokesbury and Greenmount. Foot and vehicular traffic are heavy. Cars pull up. Youth on the corner run or walk to vehicles, get money, run back to where they were standing, get a package of drugs from a partner, then run or walk to deliver goods to people waiting in cars. Usually males, ages fifteen to twenty-five, are the sellers. Buyers are males and females who are the same age and older. Sellers are African American, as are most buyers, although a few whites occasionally roll up to purchase drugs and sex.

2. Conflicting Sexual Pressures

Sex is generally for sale. In the late night, 9–11 p.m., teenage and older African American females wearing colorful, short skirts, revealing clothing, and high heel pumps walk over to parked cars or they flag cruising cars and vans. Around 1:30 a.m., older females, nineteen to twenty-one years old, with tight outfits, approach men in parked cars. They lean over, according to an observer, with "their breasts hanging out in the men's face." One puts her hand on the driver's lap. After about ten minutes of conversation, the women get in the car. However, not everyone intent on doing some tricking is successful. Nobody seems to be interested in very overweight local female prostitutes.

Many young black males have a "My baby mama drama." They profess to only be sleeping with one girl or woman. Therefore, condoms are unnecessary for them and their partner. Yet they initially appear amazed when asked: "How are you so sure she's only sleeping with you?" Then they reply with confidence: "She has no other partner."

3. Disturbing Gender Patterns

Females also sell drugs. Some have boys or older adolescent males as partners. On Barclay, between 20th and 21st Streets, a nineteen- or twenty-year-old woman complains that "some guy is going to blow my spot" by unintentionally making things hot for her (i.e., his actions would make her drug selling visible to the police and get her arrested). Some African American male youth (sixteen to twenty-four years old) have little or no respect for their African American female peers. They use abusive names for females. These males also report females place little value on themselves.

4. Minimal Parental Influence

Parental guidance and active monitoring of the target population's outside activities are seemingly non-existent. Unsupervised youth are in the street engaged in negative activities such as cursing, arguing, gambling, smoking, drinking and participating in the drug economy.

Youth report their parents are struggling with various things. Some parents get high regularly and are unable to focus on their children's lives. Others lack information about sex and HIV/AIDS to give to their children. Because some parents of the targeted youth are addicts, they do not have or teach their children adequate prevention skills. Some parents are quite concerned and constantly warn or advise their children to abstain from sexual relations and to use condoms, if they are sexually active. Other parents send children to a relative out of town or put their children in the military or some other institution to protect them. Youth are not unaware of death. They mention that not only are parents relinquishing their children, but children are also losing their parents to drugs, HIV/AIDS, abandonment, courts, prisons, homelessness, the streets and relationships.

In the summer, children under twelve years old hang out in groups of ten or more until midnight. At midnight, adult supervision of young children and adolescents is lax or non-existent. Young boys (9+ years old) play basketball in the middle of the street, roam the streets, or hang around watching their older siblings and neighborhood acquaintances. Some boys, as young as eleven years old, actively exchange money and drugs between buyers and sellers. Some older male youth play crap games.

Youth see themselves at risk for HIV/AIDS because of unprotected sex, drinking, hanging out, using drugs, and looking for a good feeling. These activities take place at peers' houses when no parent is at home as well as in school. According to one youth: "Everything from sex, the sale and use of drugs and alcohol, robbery, theft: you name it; it goes on at school."

5. Negative Environmental Influences

Major legal businesses are bars, liquor stores, carry-outs, a check cashing store, pool hall, pharmacy, hardware store, and a bail bond agency. Other institutions include churches and a recreation center.

Some sections of the community are forsaken, exposed and vacated. Approximately seventy abandoned buildings are within a two block north and south radius of Greenmount Avenue, Barclay Street from 21st to 23rd Streets, and Boone Street. Abandoned dwellings are used for sex trade, drug trade, stash houses, shooting galleries, "abandonminiums" and dumping sites. Some blocks contain uncollected trash, empty yards and parks, and abandoned houses. It is difficult to get some residents to support community development activities. Greenmount's community activism is low. Involving local churches is important. Prayer vigils are held on 24th Street and Greenmount Avenue.

There are visible and aggressive police surveillance activities at times. Marked and unmarked cars park near specific sites. A strong police presence exists at times on Barclay Street between 20th and 24th Streets. Sweeps are also conducted. Drug dealing, suspicious roaming and loitering are temporarily reduced or sent to another location or different spot on the same block. However, from one youth's perspective: "The community is held hostage by drug dealing and police searches."

The community's economic stagnation affects its social structure and interactions, and perpetuates risky behaviors. Prostitution is high in this area. On 25th Street, girls who are twelve to thirteen years old, are tricking for money to buy clothes because they cannot get jobs. "Their parents are not there for them. Sexual favors are learned and accepted behaviors. Although neighborhood drug dealing is organized, the community is not. Youth are just there, vulnerable to what pulls them (e.g., selling sex), and waiting for something to do.

Mornings (6 a.m. to 8 a.m.) are witnesses to different lifestyles. Children go to school. Adults are en route to work, dressed in suits, nurses' clothing and construction work outfits. Small-store owners open up for business. Around 7 a.m., uncustomary behavior is detectable at a house on Greenmount and 20th. According to one youth, "There is a woman on her steps reading a book. It is sad to say, but this is something unusual to see here."

6. Depressing Economic Conditions

By month's end, businesses of all types are stalled. The mood is down. Folks are simply getting by. But after midnight, those with direct deposit funds will have access to their funds. The community "seems like the calm before the storm. Activity is slow, but one can feel the anticipation for tomorrow's cash flow."

Economic and social activity resume at the month's beginning. Social service, disability and other entitlement checks hit the neighborhood. Drug sales and prostitution pick up. Money seems to be flowing. Folks come out earlier and remain out later, enjoying themselves, drinking, listening to music, playing dominoes, eating, sitting, walking, "conversating"—glad to be in another month with another dollar. "Everyone looks happy on the first of the month."

7. Inadequate Services

There are some church street ministries in the area. On the sidewalk in front of their storefront church, at Barclay and 20th Streets, several parishioners, three women and two men, preach the Word of God. A few males are in the area. No-one seems to convert or is ready to be saved. For a while, though, the people's preaching interrupts the flow of business. Service delivery is hampered by multiple issues. HIV/AIDS posters are not displayed in the community. The disease does not seem to have a visible face. Providers need a centralized way to communicate and network with other providers. City and state agencies need to adequately communicate an awareness of HIV/AIDS information and services available to special populations, e.g., the deaf community. Politicians have not adequately provided support for needed services and organizations. Providers report lack of funding and waste of existing funds. Persons working in intervention and prevention of HIV/AIDS feel highly underpaid.

Traditional methods of instructing and providing information about HIV/AIDS may not be effective for neighborhood youth. They prefer explicit manipulation of objects rather than lectures. In some mornings and afternoons, a mobile van helps residents twenty-four to forty-four years old with substance abuse, STD testing, pregnancy testing and referrals. At 10:30 a.m., two of the van's outreach workers walk up and down the street trying to talk people into coming in where there are also two HIV/AIDS counselors, a nurse practitioner and a supervisor. However, they have serious competition. On Greenmount and 21st, a young man runs by shouting "testers" (free drugs to get people hooked to buy more later). Males and females, in their early twenties, start running to get them. It is too late. All the testers are gone. Three females are highly upset. It seems like their life is over when they miss out on the tester.

Baltimore County Health Department is not seen as an institution affecting the community in any way, either as a provider of services or a place to seek help. According to one resident, "the Baltimore City Health Department is not even a part of their thought processes."

8. Competing Attitudes and Perceptions

The views youth have of their world, family, peers, the immediate community and themselves affect their willingness to participate in or refrain from risky behaviors. Living for the moment helps create a willingness to exploit themselves or others for money, sex, drugs and material possessions. Copying the behaviors of popular youth who engage in high-risk activities further endangers them.

According to service providers, some youth are concerned about contracting HIV/AIDS, but not enough to take preventive measures. Inability to read, feelings of invulnerability, absence of specific HIV/AIDS education and lack of direct experience make many youth feel HIV/AIDS is not a personal threat.

Some youth are not very concerned with contracting HIV/AIDS. However, their attitude is: "If I get the virus, then I'm going to take as many people as I can with me." Yet they are very alert about their appearance and looking "fine." From their perspective: "Looking bad almost always says HIV/AIDS." Therefore, they think anyone who has the virus should get treatment because it will make one look better.

Youth distinguish between intravenous drug users and those who use drugs in other ways. Injecting drug users are seen as more likely to have the virus. Youth think other types of drug users are almost immune. Many youth regard themselves as strong. In their minds, the virus can not or will not approach them. Many deaf persons believe HIV/AIDS is only spread to those who can hear. They lack information and services.

Some in the community regard HIV/AIDS as a moral subject, rather than a community health issue. Family members, peers and others will pass judgment about a person and how one may have become infected, rather than obtain prevention and treatment services to help individuals and reduce the spread of the virus. Moral condemnation and rumors block youth from receiving or using outreach efforts.

Testing is seen as a risky act. Some youth will not take responsibility for knowing because of guilt and fear of consequently losing social support and acceptance. One youth does not want to know if she has the virus, since people would put her away. She will no longer be loved. In her view, if she does not know, she will not have to deal with it.

Community attitudes reduce service utilization. HIV/AIDS services are not accessed partly because of stigma and peer pressure. Different types of services are needed. Youth do not use vans for testing because they are highly concerned that others may think they have HIV/AIDS.

They associate van services with junkies and people without money. Some have no idea of actual services provided by the mobile van. Youth are not aware of the role and functioning of HIV vaccines. They lack information and are wary of possible long-term effects. Youth want proof of what a vaccine is, how it works, and that it is actually safe.

Youth report that because they are black and live in certain areas, information is being withheld from them. Some think a cure exists, but "they just don't want us to have it." A few believe Magic Johnson is cured, but others disagree. No respondent is really sure. To them, a major issue is economics. Many doubt they will receive proper treatment if they become infected because they are black and low-income persons.

Drug dealing and use are seen as exciting, pleasurable, stimulating and financially lucrative. Girls, female adolescents and young women are attracted to the lifestyles of young male dealers. Possibilities of getting quick money, gifts and material possessions lure young women. Yet, in many cases, these young women must provide sex for adolescent males and men. All this increases risks of teenage pregnancies, single parenthood, Hepatitis, sexually transmitted diseases and HIV/AIDS. Coupled with alcohol use and abuse, this situation creates conditions for unprotected sexual experimentation, multiple sex partners and unsafe monogamous sexual intercourse.

What Youth Say Would Work for Them

Many Greenmount youth want alternatives that will take the attraction away from street activities. However, they lack guidance and leadership to help mobilize self-help efforts. They are also highly motivated to work on their own behalf. During conversations, focus groups and interviews, some youth also identified positive motivations. They expressed a desire for personal relief and information, readiness to take information to the rest of their community and a willingness to become empowered and respond to BCHD initiatives. They offered the following points to reduce their HIV risks:

1. Key chain condom holders help to grab people's attention and engage them in research and outreach. The distribution of condoms and literature to prostitutes, drug dealers and users can legitimate field researchers in the community. Similar efforts may help to market the Baltimore County Health Department (BCHD).

2. Informants report that removal of unnecessary red-tape and unrealistic qualifications are necessary to get general health care in Greenmount. Residents could identify other health services uptown, cross-town and downtown, but none were connected with BCHD. A community family health fair, which would include counseling, testing and health education, was seen as a useful form of entertainment and service delivery.

3. City agencies, e.g., health and sanitation, could coordinate an environmental pollution control and preservation initiative aimed at the abundance of abandoned buildings in the community. Residents maintain that the city itself could appropriately board buildings or supply materials and supervise residents as they board them.

4. Safer sex parties in a neighborhood house with respected community adults trained in HIV/AIDS are viewed as important. Youth say these settings could be used for demonstrating hands-on and/or explicit use of condoms, counseling, and pre- and post-testing.

5. Residents think community and religious groups, working with and sponsored by Baltimore's health and sanitation departments, could offer a block party as an incentive for a community clean-up. Other rewards could be free movie tickets, video games and CDs offered by merchants, pharmaceutical companies, radio stations and celebrities. One person advised: "Try to be consistent. Be out there on a constant basis, building block by block."

6. Utilizing and coordinating existing outreach services were seen as effective ways of helping the community. A directory of community-based services does not seem to exist.

7. Youth report that a van service is worthwhile and they might use it if they knew precisely what the van offered, its schedule, what takes place inside, as well as if the van's services matched the youth's after-school and evening hours. Many youth report they would use a clinic or hospital emergency room if they required HIV/AIDS prevention services.

8. Youth are not clear about treatment procedures. They also indicate a preference to be treated at home or at a clinic, emergency room or doctor's office. Rap sessions conducted by and for youth are regarded as a way to transmit and receive correct information about HIV/AIDS.

9. Youth think the spread of HIV/AIDS could be reduced by encouraging abstinence, holding focus and information groups, and through adequate messages targeted at seventeen to twenty-five-year-olds. As one person put it, "We need to meet them where they are."

10. Residents report graphic posters with harsh messages geared toward youth may help them comprehend the disease's devastating reality. Such posters

would show the pain and suffering of someone with HIV/AIDS who wants relief, but cannot find it. Teen safer-sex workshops were requested to be held at local churches, recreation centers and schools.

11. Some youth are receptive to structured discussions and questioning, and receiving or distributing condoms, literature and other outreach. Some youth want more outreach and supplies. They are receptive to receiving HIV/AIDS information and materials. However, traditional adult-oriented inducements may not motivate youth to seek information and services. Youth like activities, such as parties, which are fun. Offering gifts and monetary incentives may generate a turnout.

12. Youth and adults need an open outlet, a "sit down and release forum," to relieve themselves of a burden. Education is needed regarding how people can contract HIV/AIDS. This leads to a lack of compassion, understanding and knowledge about prevention and treatment. People do not know what to do if someone develops HIV/AIDS: Fear takes over, instead of having attitudes and skills to seek and use services. "Once you are known to be infected or have contracted the virus, it's an automatic shut-down, cut-off, shut off, as far as family members, loved ones and the community are concerned."

13. Some residents think trips by youth to an HIV/AIDS hospice would dramatically show them the reality of the epidemic and help them understand the seriousness of their risky behaviors. One explained: "We need to let them see the ugliness that may come with this disease and not just that you can live a healthy, normal life if you get tested and treated." According to a twenty-five-year-old mother, "Talking is one thing. Seeing is another. Youth take HIV for a joke, including using condoms."

14. Some older adult residents are respected as neighborhood elders and are accepted by some youth. Residences of these older residents are seen as safe houses. "Older people are treated like a neighborhood mom and dad. They have looked after them [youth] and are trusted." HIV/AIDS education and training for residents forty years and older may allow them to act as service workers for youth and be sources of safe houses.

Other adults are scorned. Some targeted youth understand they lack alternative role models whose healthy and positive behavior can be followed. On Cokesbury Street and Loch Raven, an area known for marijuana sales, a nineteen-year-old male defiantly asserted: "How are we supposed to learn from our parents if they're doing the same thing, like drinking?" Drinking appears to be a way of life for some residents. Some youth rationalize their risky activities as logical outcomes of negative adult behaviors. A typical thought of such youth is: "If they're not living their lives right, why should I?" According to one field researcher, "He knows what he's doing is wrong, but what choice does he have?" Outlets are not readily available to help them relate to and care for affected and infected family members. Discussions about HIV/AIDS are rare and socially uncomfortable. According to one person, "The conversation we were having is not an acceptable conversation in the community."

Amidst what we observed were encouraging moments. One Saturday night, a party of drug ex-users lets out, but folks do not want to leave the scene. Over one hundred people congregate. Cars are double-parked. Talk and interaction are wholesome, supportive and uplifting. There are many stories of how long people have been clean and descriptions of accomplishments since they have been off drugs. According to an observer, "It was very inspirational." The scene lasts for over an hour. Such moments may be duplicated with emulation stories by former users and possibly dealers, street walkers, persons living with the virus, and affected loved ones. Community-based businesses or other institutions could be asked to sponsor and/or be the site of a similar gathering.

Recommendations

There are six major recommendations, each of which is accompanied by suggested strategies for curtailing the epidemic.

1. Provide Coordinated Community-based HIV/AIDS Services during Non-Traditional Hours.

Strategies

- Train teams of health educators and street outreach workers who will specifically focus on targeted areas during non-traditional hours.
- Van service should be routinely present and available on demand.

2. Develop, Structure, Mobilize and Support Community-based Initiatives.

Strategies

- Organize safer-sex parties and community health fairs at recreation centers and other venues.
- Coordinate church and other faith-based initiatives to develop, assess and deliver messages of risk reduction, prevention and treatment.
- Saturate the community with a wide range of useful, relevant and practical information and materials. Provide bulletin boards and information not only about HIV/AIDS, but also about events and topics of interest to the targeted age category. Baltimore City Health Department should make information, supplies and services available. "To make it available, to have the choice to use it, is a shot of hope for the community," according to one person.
- Select and train community residents to maintain neighborhood safe-houses containing useful information, supplies and referral sources.
- Rehabilitate and use vacated properties to provide more and better community-based services.

3. Provide Comprehensive and Specialized Services.

Strategies

- Outreach teams should address such needs as parenting classes, sex education, budgeting, job readiness, vocational training, GED preparation, and family and peer relationships.
- Police should play a greater role in strengthening the community. There should be more street officers, and they should be a source of information and resources. Officers should be educated to communicate about the basic facts of HIV/AIDS and where to get help.
- Enhance drug treatment to include preventing HIV/AIDS and rehabilitating the person, as well as treating the addiction.
- Provide adequate funding for workers' salaries and health care facilities.
- Baltimore City Health Department should have its workers walk the beats to establish links with residents, assess their needs and provide appropriate services.

4. Hold Neighborhood Forums for Communication and Assistance.

Strategies

- A community-based support group for youth and other family members is needed for prevention and treatment.
- Persons who are HIV-infected or have HIV/AIDS should be invited to a forum in the community. One would be a person who is apparently doing relatively well and the other who is not. Persons living with HIV/AIDS and role-playing are needed to show residents the many things one has to do to maintain a healthy and productive lifestyle while living with HIV/AIDS. For example, demonstrate the strict frequency and number of medicines one has to take. The other role-player or actual person with HIV/AIDS could be one who is shunned by family and loved ones, and is not living a healthy or productive lifestyle. For example, demonstrate consequences of being ostracized.
- Fund a consultant to generate meetings, and to obtain and stay on top of updated information.

5. Provide Continuous, Appropriate, Attractive and Persuasive Information and Messages.

Strategies

- Television and other media attractive to youth should be used for attention-getting facts and points.

- A youth-sensitive and targeted counseling and testing marathon should be initiated.
- Health staff should be trained to share information in a way that is readily acceptable to youth. People need to be comfortable when receiving services. Baltimore City Health Department should conduct on-going seminars, hold focus groups and distribute information.

6. Mobilize and Work with Responsive Community Youth.

Strategies

- New community leadership needs to be developed from among youth. People report they know best what works for them. Governmental bureaucracy and funds should not be depended on, but used as a source of technical assistance.
- Technical assistance is needed to help develop a collective of youth, parents, religious institutions and schools.
- Create a peer education unit to help develop and mobilize peer buddies and older partner networks. Provide them with correct and current information and materials that are sensitive to the targeted population.

Conclusion

A weakened political economy and community de-stabilization contribute to the spread of HIV/AIDS, and an inadequate response from public health officials. The contraction and transmission of HIV/AIDS take place in inter-related contexts of social relations, perceptions, socially constructed realities, attitudes, cognition, feelings, skills and behaviors. Prevention and treatment efforts are linked to issues of power, history, political economy, identity and culture, and interactions with race, ethnicity, class and gender (Quimby and Friedman 2003). In the mix are real human beings with day-to-day survival concerns. They are not sociological statistics, political abstractions or bureaucratic things. Certain neighborhoods in Baltimore City, Maryland, have been politically and economically abandoned, neglected, and thrust into a parallel, underground economy and social system. They have their own norms, values, lifestyles, concerns, problems, acceptable solutions, definitions of normal, and conceptions of deviance.

In Greenmount, East Baltimore, the level and types of knowledge about HIV/AIDS are dismal. Two decades into the epidemic the myths persist, e.g., the virus can be spread by touching an infected person or by sharing cigarettes. On the street, in homes, among peers and loved ones, tenacious moral judgments and readiness to accuse or defend help propel ignorance and misinformation. Rather than be tested, for some persons it is preferable to risk death and physical suffering than endure the humiliation and rejection that may come with the social knowledge that one is infected. Denial and avoidance become survival strategies to ensure social acceptance. There are consequences of perceived inaction: not having sex, declining to drink, choosing not to do drugs and not having the momentary fun or participating in the lucrative lure of the corner drug trade. These consequences may be considerably more immediately than using a condom. The installed goals are getting high, designer clothes, cash, admiration, status, recognition, respect, entrepreneurship, excitement and being dread.

Youth in East Baltimore, like those elsewhere, are driven by a desire for pleasure, identity, self-worth, respect, acceptance, power, prestige and wealth. Yet, a collapsed inner-city economy and bankrupt educational system provide few perceived resources and opportunities for authentic employment, social mobility and a meaningful existence. Objectively, high-risk behaviors make people more vulnerable to contracting or spreading HIV/AIDS. Yet, subjectively, high-risk can also mean actions that expose people to a loss of their ability to socially control their social world. In this sense, commercial sex work may be an attempt to reduce the 'high-risks' of poverty. Female prostitution can be a job and a perceived means of self-empowerment, e.g., to feed one's children and oneself, to minimize economic dominance by a male, to earn money to buy basic necessities and luxury items. Moreover, according to this sensibility, not getting high is risky. Getting high may lead to death, but for now its sensations nullify the pain of rejection.

In Greenmount, many adolescent females and younger girls are enticed by seductive charms, promises and deliverance of material goods for sex. Young boys hang out with and watch older youth. The cliques and lifestyle are appealing, but require admission. Entrance tickets are stamped: willingness to use alcohol and/or other drugs, consensual and unprotected sex, multiple sex partners, loyalty to the group, active participation in or approval of dealing in drugs and commercial sex, and an assumption of personal invulnerability or that HIV/AIDS is secondary, unless it hits close to home.

Social and personal reactions to HIV/AIDS often include uninformed moral condemnation, fear and ostracism, rather than compassionate and supportive treatment-seeking behaviors. Moreover, factual information, wellness, prevention, health maintenance and treatment are seemingly hard to obtain. Many youth cannot identify formal health services in their area, but can reference those outside. They think their community is neglected because of race and class. Some assert that a cure for HIV/AIDS already exists, but that it is not being shared. They are wary of participating in vaccine trials because of insufficient information about the vaccines.

Hence, mobilizing around HIV/AIDS is a difficult task. Yet youth are not unconscious or lethargic. When asked about their needs and suggestions, many are eager to respond and share their thoughts. They reveal a need to express themselves and relieve their fears about HIV/AIDS and discuss reliable, current information. Structured, ongoing community forums are requested to stimulate and maintain community awareness and involvement. Some youth report a readiness and desire to receive youth-oriented HIV/AIDS advertisements, featuring rappers and other respected and emulated people. Such youth report not only a desire to receive information and services, but the necessity for community development. They request workshops on community mobilizing, fundraising and leadership training. For them, the major modes of transmitting the virus are unprotected sexual intercourse, drug use and a lifestyle almost compelled by living in a vulnerable community which tolerates risky behaviors. Reducing them requires community construction and defense. According to some youth in East Baltimore, HIV/AIDS is a disease which requires individual and community responses. As one person put it "We have talked to several youths who are ready, willing and able. They just need to know when and where."

Public Policy Implications

Two public policy implications are offered here. First, dismissal of recommendations by community residents amounts to continued sentences of death and disability. Although RARE in Baltimore was a community-based technical assistance strategy, it was not structured to be accountable to the community. To be effective, public health programs require community participation in planning, implementing and evaluating response strategies. This includes meaningful involvement in site selection, data collection and analysis, interpretation of findings, and planning, implementing and evaluating interventions.

Second, sustained public health campaigns must be rooted in collaborative and cooperative partnerships that respond to issues that are regarded as more meaningful than those defined by official authorities. Failure to adequately and comprehensively address structural and cultural matters of consequence has the potential for launching programs that are deemed irrelevant by targeted residents.

References

AYPF (1997) *What's Really Happening with America's Out-of-School Youth? Washington*: American Youth Policy Forum.

BSAS (2003) Smart Steps, Treating Baltimore's Drug Problem. Baltimore Substance Abuse Systems, Inc. Available at http://www.drugstrategies.org/Index.html. Accessed 16, 2003.

CDC. (1999) *HIV AIDS Surveillance Reports*. Atlanta: Centers for Disease Con trol and Prevention.

CDC. (2000) *HIV AIDS Surveillance Reports*. Atlanta: Centers for Disease Control and Prevention.

CDC. (1998) *Trends in the HIV and AIDS Epidemic*. Atlanta: Centers for Disease Control and Prevention.

HHS (2000) *Healthy People 2010*. Washington: U.S. Department of Health and Human Services.

HHS (1999) HHS announces three sites for special crisis response teams to battle HIV/AIDS in minority communities. [press release]. U.S. Department of Health and Human Services; June 16.

Institute of Medicine (2002) *Unequal Treatment: Confronting Racial and Ethnic Disparities in Health Care*. Washington: National Academy Press.

JOTF (1999) *Baltimore's Choice: Workers & Jobs for a Thriving Economy and U.S. Census: 1998 Income Reported in the March 1999 Current Population Survey*. Baltimore: Job Opportunities Task Force.

Quimby, E., Friedman, S.R. (2003) Dynamics of Black Mobilization against AIDS in New York City. In P. Conrad and V. Leiter (eds.), *Health and Health Care as Social Problems* (pp. 145–159). Lanham, MD: Rowman & Littlefield.

NCJJ (2003) *National Juvenile Court Data Archive*. Washington: National Center for Juvenile Justice.

Needle, H.R., Trotter, II, R.T., Singer, M., et al. (2003) Rapid Assessment of the HIV/AIDS Crisis in Racial and Ethnic Minority Communities: An Approach for Timely Community Interventions. *American Journal of Public Health*, 93: 970–979.

PSCS (2002). *Informational Brochure*. Maryland Division of Parole and Probation, Department of Public Safety & Correctional Services.

Smith, V., Steele, J.J. (2003). Snapshots of the Greatest City in America. Baltimore City Paper, January 22–28.

Trotter, R.T., Needle, H.R. (1999) *Crisis Response Teams and Communities Combat HIV/AIDS in Racial and Ethnic Minority Populations: Rapid Assessment, Rapid Response, and Evaluation Field Assessment Training Workbook*. Washington: Office of HIV/AIDS Policy, U.S. Department of Health and Human Services.

U.S. Census Bureau (1998) *Statistical Abstract of the United States*. Washington: U.S. Census Bureau.

U.S. Census Bureau (2001) *Challenges and Policy Options: Labor Market Conditions among 16–24 Year Old Adults in Maryland and the Baltimore PMSA*. Washington: U.S. Census Bureau.

Chapter 6

AIDS in Philadelphia: Emerging from the Shadow of Crack

William Eric Perkins
David Metzger

Introduction

The Philadelphia RARE Advisory Group met in August 1999 to initiate the process and identify target populations. The group decided to target two specific zip-code areas, 19104 in West Philadelphia and 19140 in North Philadelphia. These two areas had a significant number of new AIDS cases reported through March 31, 1999. Based upon AIDS case data, observations of the Advisory Group, and recent data from seroincidence studies, it was further specified that crack-smoking women would be the specific targeted focus of the field team's research.

The Philadelphia field team was selected by the Advisory Group and the team co-leaders were selected in consultation with the Office of HIV/AIDS Policy of Health and Human Services and the City of Philadelphia Department of Health. The field team was led by Dr. David Metzger, Director of the Opiate/AIDS Division of the Center for Studies of Addiction at the University of Pennsylvania of Pennsylvania Health System, and Dr. William Eric Perkins, Senior Research Scholar with the African American Literacy and Culture Project at the University of Pennsylvania. Field team members came from a wide variety of outreach, counseling, referral, and treatment facilities and services.

Once the field team was assembled, it was divided into two subteams, one for North Philadelphia and one for West Philadelphia. The full team was trained in August of 1999, and began its work on September 8. Data were collected through December 3, 1999. Weekly team meetings were held throughout this process to analyze data and schedule new data collection activities, develop outreach strategies, and engage in serious deliberations about the risk behaviors and what might constitute meaningful and appropriate interventions.

A report of the preliminary findings and proposed action plan with detailed recommendations was presented by the field team to the HIV/AIDS Advisory Board on December 20, 1999. This chapter includes a detailed description of the target areas and populations, the methods used by the field team and the team's findings. Recommendations for intervention are designed to be not only necessary but achievable and sustainable. They reflect the collective judgment of the field team and incorporate feedback from the Advisory Board. As Philadelphia moves into its third decade of the AIDS epidemic, strategies of prevention and care must remain responsive to the needs and sensitivities of those most affected.

Background

AIDS and Race in Philadelphia

In Philadelphia, AIDS has had a disproportionate impact on African Americans and Latinos. The most recent census data indicate that Philadelphia has a total population of approximately 1,451,372. Of these, 617,065 (42.5%) are African American and 60,379 (4%) are Latino, Asian, and other minorities.

Since the first diagnosis of AIDS in Philadelphia in 1981, through October of 1999, 12,353 individuals in the city have been diagnosed with AIDS. Of these, 7,040 (64%) were African American and 1,171 (11 %) were of other minorities. Thus, while minorities account for 47% of the total population in Philadelphia, 75% of the diagnosed AIDS cases are among African Americans and other minorities.

The "AIDS disparity gap" between whites and minorities is widening. Between January 1 and September 30 of 1999, 1,071 individuals were diagnosed with AIDS. Of these 733 (68%) were African American and 134 (12.6%) were of other minorities.

Risk Groups and Race

The disproportionate ethnic impact can be found in each of the three populations at primary risk for AIDS—men who have sex with men (MSM), injection drug users (IDUs) and heterosexuals.

MSMs

Since 1981, 5,157 men who have sex with men have been diagnosed with AIDS. Of these, 59% (3,028) were African American or Latino. Between January 1 and September 30, 1999, African Americans and Latinos accounted for 58% of MSMs diagnosed with AIDS.

IDUs

Of the 3,155 injection drug users (IDUs) diagnosed with AIDS since 1981, 2,738 (87%) were African American or Latino. During the last reporting period, between January 1 and September 30, 1999, African Americans and Latinos accounted for 87% of IDUs diagnosed with AIDS.

Heterosexuals

Of the 1,577 heterosexuals diagnosed with AIDS since the beginning of the epidemic in Philadelphia, 90% (1423) were African American or Latino. Between January 1 and September 30, 1999, African Americans and Latinos accounted for 91% of heterosexuals diagnosed with AIDS.

AIDS cases are growing most rapidly among heterosexuals, further complicating the disproportionate impact of AIDS on African Americans and Latinos in Philadelphia. Data reflected in the chart below from 1999 indicate that AIDS diagnoses among heterosexuals have shown a dramatic increase. While this may reflect changes in reporting, it may also be an indication of a shift in the predominate mode of transmission and increase in populations at risk.

Target Areas

As noted, two zip codes, 19140 and 19104, were designated as the target areas of assessment. The area of 19140 is located in North Philadelphia and zip code 19104 is located in West Philadelphia. Within each area, the team identified smaller areas in which drug sales, drug use, and sex work are concentrated. Early in the process these areas were labeled "risk pockets" by the field team and are shown as the shaded areas in the following map. The risk pocket in 19104 extends into the zip code areas of 19139 and 19131.

The Bottom

As can be seen in the following map, the West Philadelphia risk pocket is bounded by 39th Street to the east and 49th Street to the west, and lies between Westminster Avenue to the north and Merideth Street to the south. This area is known locally as "the Bottom." The Bottom is bisected by Lancaster Avenue and is best described as an aging, densely populated, residential area.

Hunting Park

The 19140 risk pocket is bounded by West Hunting Park Avenue to the North, Germantown Avenue to the west, Luzerne and Butler Streets to the South, and 9th Street to the east. The area includes the lower half of Hunting Park which gives the area its name. Broad Street is the major thoroughfare.

Target Area Profiles

Unfortunately, the most current and complete socio-economic data for the target areas are data from the 1990 Census. Despite the age of these data, the following summaries are reported to highlight the demographic characteristics of the areas and the long-term nature of their current economic distress.

Table 6.1: Risk Area Demographics

	The Bottom	Hunting Park
Population (1990):	19,301	18,583
Area:	1 sq. mi.	1 sq. mi.
Race: Black	18,736 (97%)	9,256 (49%)
White	396 (2%)	1,563 (8%)
Latino/a	80 (<1%)	7,764 (42%)
Unoccupied Housing Units:	1,578 (26%)	901(15%)
% Employed:	79%	84%
Household Income (med):	$13,174	$16,430
% Below Poverty Level:	7%	36%

Source: U.S. Census of Population, 1993.

The Bottom, in West Philadelphia, is an area of less than one square mile in size. The vast majority (97%) of its residents are African American. Although a very high rate (26%) of the housing units were unoccupied in 1990, it is estimated that this rate has dramatically increased over the past 10 years. Thirty-seven percent of the residents of this area were living below the poverty level and the median household income for this area was $13,174 in 1990. This is slightly more than one-half the median household income ($25,176) for the city as a whole.

The Hunting Park risk pocket in North Philadelphia is characterized by a high degree of poverty, unemployment, and abandoned properties. In the 1990 Census, median household income for the three census tracts which define this risk pocket (197,198, and 203) was $16,430, slightly more than 50% of the median household income for all of Philadelphia during the same time period. The proportion of people living below the poverty level in the year before the 1990 Census was 36%. Among those in the labor force the unemployment rate was 16%. In 1989, 15% of the housing units were not occupied.

Methods

Three classes of respondents were targeted for data collection. These three respondent groups were labeled by the team as 1) community experts, 2) community leaders, and 3) service providers. Community experts refer to those individuals with knowledge of the target area—residents, sex workers, drug dealers, and others encountered during street outreach activities. Community leaders refer to those individuals who are knowledgeable about the target area and who have a formal leadership role in the community: police, religious leaders, and leaders of community organizations. Service providers were program administrators and staff of agencies providing HIV-prevention services to the target area.

Four qualitative methods, discussed below, were used in the collection of data for the RARE process in Philadelphia:

Street Interviews

To more effectively collect data from community experts and members of our primary target population—crack-smoking women—the field team used a modified interview strategy. This particular adaptation of RARE methodology is a synthesis of the formal, lengthy interview with the "street intercept" method. Using mini-cassette tape recorders, field team members were able to record interviews with community experts with minimal intrusion into their activities. Interviews were often conducted while respondents were engaged in the search for potential tricks or on a "mission" (acquiring the next hit of crack cocaine). It would not have been feasible to conduct a more formal interview in a private setting.

Individual Interviews

Individual interviews were used to collect information from people with whom private sessions could be scheduled. These included community experts, community leaders and service providers. The interviews were conducted using a semi-structured interview format. The questions were designed to document the respondents' familiarity with the risk pocket, their perception of drug sales and use in the area, their understanding of HIV risk and their ideas regarding needed services. With the awareness and consent of the respondent, these interviews were tape recorded and transcribed.

Focus Groups

The field team utilized focus groups to elaborate on team observations and the reports from individual interviews. Focus groups were held with clients in a drug treatment program, with individuals receiving services from a prevention program, and community experts from the target areas. The focus groups were also tape recorded and transcribed. The focus groups used modified versions of the interview guidelines to structure the group discussion.

Observation and Assessment

Observation and assessment were ongoing activities for the RARE field team. Following an initial training in the strategies for safe and effective street outreach, team members conducted regular visits to the target areas. Team members were expected to work in small groups and carry fliers that explained the RARE process. Visits were scheduled to take place on various days each week throughout the ten week data collection phase. The primary objective of this method was to become familiar with the population and document the patterns and locations of activity in each area. Many of the street interviews described above took place during these observation visits. Team members also photographed key locations associated with risky behavior. Observations took place throughout the day and night. The field team met weekly to review findings and to discuss implications for prevention.

As shown in the following table, during the ten-week data collection phase, the field team accumulated over four hundred hours of observation, and completed sixty street interviews, forty individual interviews and six focus groups.

Table 6.2: Summary of Hours and Interviews

	Experts	Leaders	Providers
Observations	200 hrs	200 hrs	50 hrs
Street Interviews	30	20	10
Individual Interviews	10	20	10
Focus Groups	14	12	

Through weekly debriefing and discussion sessions, team members synthesized observations, interview findings and experiences. Four prevention relevant themes emerged and were reinforced by redundancies in the data. These included: 1) the observation of concentrated areas of risk; 2) the widespread lack of accurate and complete information on HIV transmission, prevention, and prevalence; 3) the high rate of "mixing" that occurs in these risk pockets; and 4) the numerous barriers to consistent condom use. Each of these four findings is described in detail below with representative excerpts from interview and focus group transcripts.

Findings

Risk Pockets

Our field teams found in each target geographic area (blocks and groups of blocks) locations with high concentrations of individuals involved in exchange of sex for drugs or money. The most common drug exchanged was crack cocaine. These locations also had numerous drug sales, indoor and out-door spaces where drugs can be used, abandoned houses interspersed with occupied housing, and neglected open spaces. We have labeled these areas risk pockets. As reflected in this respondent's statement, sex exchanges occur around the clock in the risk pocket.

> Respondent 01: I used to see them; they'll be on the corner say Jerome Street. They'll be on the corner any time from way in the morning like eight until the next morning. I used to work hours from 6:00 to 2:30 in the morning. Sometimes when I walked home from the bus and that wasn't often, but when I did, I would see that they would be on the corner doing their business.

Both risk pockets have a large number of abandoned properties and neglected spaces allowing risk behaviors to become embedded in the landscape.

> Respondent 05: Look at the grass over there, right over there by the telephone pole. Man, it looks like a war zone over there. It's not supposed to be like that. That area is supposed to be a park, you know what I mean? It keeps a lot of elderly people from walking through and kids from playing. You can't play out there; they cleaned up some hypodermic needles the other day right around the corner. I sweep from here all the way around by my alley way. I cleaned up about three or four hypodermic needles on the ground. My children, when they come, my grandkids, they playing, riding their bicycles.

> They might fall on one of those things or the glass around here. You know what I'm trying to say?

As depicted in the following statement from a resident in the Hunting Park area, there are many people living in these risk pockets who are committed to the neighborhood and want to see things improve.

> Respondent 02: I've been in this neighborhood approximately ten years. It was as far as I know always a family-oriented block. I had some friends who lived here and there was always children playing ten years ago, twenty years ago and even now. I like the block, but it is rapidly deteriorating. My property value has probably decreased by ten thousand dollars because right next to my home there are four abandoned properties, across the street from me directly there's an abandoned property, to left and across the street there's two abandoned properties; but I'm not going anywhere.

The prevalence and visibility of drug sales and sex work contribute to a sense of abandonment and loss of control.

> Okay. I'm from down the Bottom. I'm from around the corner of 46th St. What I know is: they sell all kinds of drugs around there. Yeah, well, I trick a lot, and it's really totally out of hand because they disrespect the women. I have seen in crack houses people have orgies. I have seen girls do guys. I have seen a lot and it's really out of hand.

Through extensive observation and interviews, the field team was able to gain an understanding of the patterns of risk in each pocket. Risk pattern refers to the interaction between location, time of day, type of sex exchange and risk group. This level of detail provides an opportunity to design highly specific prevention intervention.

After carefully noting the time of day when high-risk groups were publicly assessable, it is very clear that there is virtually a complete mismatch between the times when prevention and care activities are available and when people who engage in HIV high-risk behaviors are most active and assessable. The vast majority of crack users and sex trades stay off the streets during the day when services are available and are most active at night when services are not available.

Street Science: Facts, Misinformation and Mythology

HIV risk and prevention were not well understood by the community experts that we interviewed on the streets. Often their knowledge of HIV included a mixture of facts, misinformation and mythology. We call this cultural information "street science." Yet, community experts appeared quite interested in new information and amenable to altering their conceptions under one condition: the information has to be delivered by trusted sources that are respected by their community. Heath Department reports and other "official" data do not meet this test. The following community expert (a drug dealer) reveals both a level of awareness of treatments for AIDS as well as an unconventional view of the HIV epidemic.

> Respondent 03: Well, anybody's at risk for HIV, not only in this area, any area. It seems to me honestly, the more money you got the more that AIDS shit come about. Yeah, there's people off in corners that don't have the medical insurance and shit like that, the drug cocktails and all of that, to take for their AIDS. But, you best believe them fucking rich people are getting that shit 'cause they got the money; so they can try and do anything they fucking want to do.
>
> If you look at that shit on a worldwide scale, and I just was reading that Dow Jones report like a month or two ago, more people with money get that shit then (give it to) ghetto people. Because the more people with the dough, they're liable to try any mother fucking thing and they're trying anything and sleeping with anybody.

The following excerpt reflects the degree to which the government is perceived as an agent in the drug trade, influencing the types and availability of drugs on the street. This respondent also goes on to minimize the risk associated with crack.

> Respondent: I think all the drug dealers that have the bad shit should be locked up. Don't lock up the ones that have the good shit. Lock up the nasty ass poison ass shit...the government knows 'cause they probably get the good shit in the country. They're the ones, they got the best scientist, the best chemist; they the ones that give us the bad shit. And why is it, hold on, why is it, okay, now check this out, why is it powder? Back in the day, there was one kind of cocaine. One powder was for everybody. You can shot it, snort it or smoke it right. How come, all of a sudden now, they got snorting drugs, shooting drugs and smoking drugs. . . . I think the safest way to do, the safest drug in world is to smoke crack because you (only) need baking soda.

In the following segment, we hear a series of common myths about HIV transmission and the role of the government in allowing the epidemic to continue.

> Subj01: Everybody, everybody in this whole world is (having sex). I think they doing it (transmitting HIV) with a bug. I think there's a bug somewhere, they (the government) gave it to a bug and the bug come, like a mosquito, that's how they did it. I'm saying everyone in the whole world (can get it), it might be in the air, airborne, know what I mean. I'm saying how come some people get it and others don't. It might be the mood the

person is in, or something. . . . Condoms and bleach don't work. Why is the Health Department telling people that I can use needles and then you bleach them out? What's up with that? Why is the Health Department doin it?

(Furthermore) Why they putting out a myth that bleach is actually gonna change something airborne?. . . . The air has a better chance of killing the virus than bleach. The bleach ain't gonna do nothing. So why they givin' out (lies)? They know what they doin'. Part of the concern is just like Vietnam; it's a plague that the government is a part of. It would never be like this; it would never got this far. You know what I mean? It ain't about the homosexual community that they credit or the drug community. It's economic based, to get rid of a number of people because the welfare roles and the drug programs because it cuts (down) HMO (costs) and hospitalization—the whole nine yards.

Mixing

One of the defining epidemiologic features of the risk pocket is the high level of sexual interaction that takes place among individuals. This interaction often occurs among individuals from diverse geographic areas, socio-economic and ethnic backgrounds, drug use patterns and histories, sexual preferences and health statuses. As a result, the probability of viral transmission and spread across groups is greatly increased. As highlighted in the following series of quotes from respondents, the team repeatedly heard reports about people from different areas of the city and suburbs attracted to the risk pockets by the availability of sex. The availability of sex attracts heterosexuals, gays and bisexuals alike.

Interviewer: Who do you think that the girls talk to? What kind of guys?

Subj03: White guys, black guys, Chinese guys; all types of shit be coming through here.

Interviewer: Is it a drive through?

Subj03: Indian guys.

Interviewer: Do they walk up to them?

Subj03: They drive more than a lot, 90%, 99% of them drive.

Male: I'm an addict. I've been active in addiction for twenty-seven years. I first got into tricking because I'm a homosexual and I had a very unsatisfactory relationship for twenty years and the last five of them, I was having no sex with my lover. And, um, I found that when I was out at the crack houses there are men in crack houses that will do just about anything for drugs, just as there are women that will do anything for the drugs. And, ah, I used to offer the dealers blow jobs when I ran out of money, and I

> felt I was getting one over on them because I was homosexual and they didn't know it and I was enjoying myself or so I thought.
>
> Female: I got friends who deal with men but have women also. I guess they call it like being bisexual—like having that closet life so they won't spook family members and their friends. Especially if they decide that they interested in (a woman). They go both (ways).
>
> I've been a heroin addict for like I started thirty-five years ago. From when the AIDS epidemic first started in the early 80s, I was on the path. I'm a highly sexed person and like to see the tricks out on Broad Street. . . They'd get me to drive them around; they wanted a place to sit in the winter time and thaw off. So you know I was there. So you know it was like free sex with them. Since then people come in the neighborhood that don't live here looking for tricks or looking for the drugs.

Condom Use

Condoms are not consistently used in these risk pockets. While some sex workers stated that they require condoms for all of their partners, all respondents reported some circumstances in which condoms would not be used. The decision is based foremost upon the apparent risk posed by a partner or a potential partner. Familiarity is a key factor in making the decision to use or request that a condom be used. The following excerpt reflects some of the disadvantages of condom use that sex workers encounter.

> Sex Worker: It's to our disadvantage; the lubricated ones taste like shit, okay, that shit tastes worse then cum itself, that shit tastes nasty. You don't have the green ones all the time, all that shit tastes really, really, really, really nasty, nasty ass taste in your mouth but for most men, it's psychological. I'm at the point where they'll take them off or they'll come inside of it and then say, see they play games with condoms.

The following passage highlights the inconsistency of condom use among individuals in relationships even when fully aware of their partner's risk status.

> Male Interviewer: Without you saying no names or saying your name, do you have sex with one of the girls in the park?
>
> Subj02: Very rarely.
>
> Male Interviewer: Have you ever?
>
> Subj02: Yeah.
>
> Male Interviewer: When you did, did you have, did you use protection?
>
> Subj02: Um, sometimes.

Male Interviewer: Sometimes; has it been all the time?

Subj02: Use protection all the time? No.

Male Interviewer: Tell me your reason why you didn't use protection.

Subj02: We were in a relationship.

Male Interviewer: Was she messing with anybody else that you know of?

Sub/02: Yeah.

Male Interviewer: She was and that didn't matter to you?

Subj02: Well, I mean you know uh it did, but apparently it didn't.

Recommendations

Recommendation 1: A street-level HIV education campaign needs to be conducted in each of the risk pockets.

This campaign should highlight the risk behaviors associated with the sex-for-crack economy. It must be integrated into the risk pocket with messages delivered by community members who are respected by the target population and use acceptable and accessible media. The team found serious distrust of what is perceived as official information. Messages about HIV communicated through the "official media" are held in suspicion. Although HIV was not seen as a high priority issue for those at risk, the field team found substantial interest among risk takers in learning more about the epidemic.

Recommendation 2: Low-threshold, saturated (LTS) prevention intervention should be instituted in each risk pocket.

LTS interventions would be rooted in the community and have the goal of providing access to prevention related services and supplies to these risk pockets. Many community experts were unaware of current HIV, prevention initiatives and methods for accessing existing services. Prevention services and prevention supplies are typically not available during evening, night time and weekend hours. HIV risk is a multi-dimensional problem related to a wide variety of socio-economic factors for which existing service systems are in place, but do not penetrate these risk pockets.

> Recommendation 3: Risk pockets can be found throughout the city and the RARE process should be used to assist in targeting and evaluating public health and prevention services.

Existing HN prevention outreach workers in Philadelphia should be educated and oriented to the RARE methodology. At this stage of the HIV epidemic in Philadelphia, a substantial amount of HIV risk appears to be concentrated in small geographic clusters. These small risk pockets increase the potential for mixing and viral transmission and can become the focus of public health intervention.

> Recommendation 4: There is need for an Inter-Agency Task Force composed of appropriate representatives from agencies that have as their charge serving the target populations.

Task Force representatives should come from the Housing Authority, the School District, Human Services, the Health Department and the criminal justice system. Coordination of the Task Force's activities would be by the Low-Threshold, Saturated (LTS) team in each intervention zone. Many of the field team's observations concerned the paucity of services in the two intervention zones. Social services and health-related services seem to have bypassed these areas. Arresting the spread of the virus in these two zones will require strong coordinated effort by the entire health, social service and criminal justice establishment.

Chapter 7

AIDS in the Shadow of Power: Washington, D.C.

Ernest Quimby
Arvilla Payne-Jackson

Why Washington?

The AIDS epidemic began in Washington, D.C., with fourteen diagnosed AIDS cases among whites, seven among blacks and only one Hispanic case in 1982. By 1988, blacks led in new diagnosed cases with five hundred fifty to whites total of four hundred fifty-seven, and Hispanics thirty-four. By 1999, there were six hundred ninety-nine new AIDS cases among blacks to one hundred forty-eight whites, whose rates were in decline since 1993, and fifty-nine Hispanics. This is a 27% increase for blacks in ten years and forty-nine fold increase since 1982. What is unique about Washington, D.C., in the AIDS epidemic is that there is no backdrop of deindustrialization and urban job flight to drive an epidemic of drug trafficking and abuse as was the case in other AIDS epicenters. Work in government and in related District services has been a growth industry for decades. So it may be surprising that the District's AIDS epidemic looks very similar to the epidemic in other cities.

Washington, D.C., may not appear different because the vast majority of AIDS cases in the initial years were among gay-identified and bisexual men who worked in Washington's many government bureaus and other offices. By 1988, black gay-identified males took and maintained the lead in diagnosed cases (462) over their white and Hispanic counterparts. The number of AIDS cases among black gay men nearly tripled over the next six years before beginning a gradual decrease. The number of cases among bisexual males or men who do not gay-identify and who have sex with other men and women was consistently the highest for black males between 1982 and 1999; the number of reported cases reached a peak in 1993 at two hundred twenty-five for blacks, sixty-five for whites and fourteen for Hispanics. Since 1993, the numbers have gradually decreased each year to ninety cases for blacks, forty for whites and twelve for Hispanics in 1999.

Since 1994, the AIDS epidemic in Washington, D.C., has shown evidence of expansion to the larger heterosexual population. AIDS cases among heterosexual adult/adolescent males and pediatric males steadily increased from one reported case in 1982 to a high of six hundred thirty-nine in 1994, five hundred thirty-three of whom were black, eighty-two white and twenty-four Hispanic—29.7% of all cases. By 1999 the number of cases had dropped to three hundred seventy-seven, of which two hundred ninety-nine were black, sixty white, and twenty-five Hispanic. But the heterosexual proportion of all cases had increased to 41.6% of all new AIDS cases. Among new AIDS cases, black women have consistently had proportionately higher numbers of cases than either white or Hispanic women since 1984. Within this context of a still evolving AIDS epidemic, RARE was conducted. It was a pioneering and innovative adaptation of timely research and technical assistance methods which have been applied in varied settings (Manderson and Aaby 1992; Scrimshaw and Hurtado 1987; Stimpson, et al. 1998).

Beginning a RARE Project

As in other cities (HHS, 1999; Needle et al. 2003; Trotter and Needle 1999; Watts and Lewis 2000), the mayor requested federal financial and logistical assistance to better understand the city's AIDS epidemic. After approval from the Office of AIDS, District health officials met with the field team and federal officials. An advisory committee was organized, and met in October 2000, and decided which areas of the District to target. Two ethnographers were hired to direct the research, assessment and evaluation.

The Sites

Four sites were selected from the District's eight wards. The advisory committee selected each site because they represented different populations with vulnerability to the AIDS epidemic. Site 1 is an ethnic mixture of black, white and Latino homosexuals. Site 2 has a large population of Africans and Caribbean ethnic groups of which little is known. Site 3 is predominantly African American with limited available services. Site 4 was selected because of its high incidence of heterosexual female and pediatric AIDS cases.

Despite Washington's lack of a labor-intensive industrial job base, African Americans historically, and in more recent years Hispanics, have been attracted to the city's service industries. As in other U.S. cities, suburbanization and white flight left large tracts of substantial central-city housing for lower income and racially segregated blacks.

Notwithstanding its steady job-base and economic revitalization in the 1990s, some District neighborhoods remained in poverty. As businesses and elected political leaders developed the city's downtown business and tourist areas, infrastructural development of working class and poor neighborhoods was neglected. Despite assurances, the construction of a convention center did not result in promised trickle-down economics of job training, employment, neighborhood entrepreneurship and community development. The District's only public hospital closed. Public school performance remained sub-par. Emergent gentrification aggravated structural conditions for economically and politically marginalized residents, characterized by rapid rises in land values, dramatic increases in rent and housing costs, residential displacement, loss of community institutions and reduced public services. Downtown redevelopment and emergent gentrification of nearby areas coincided with race and class. A greater proportion of residents' earnings and fixed public income was paid for health care. Consequently, African Americans and Latinos in outlying neighborhoods demanded living wages, affordable revitalization, stabilization of their communities, quality and accessible health care, direct participation in planning and decision-making, better schools, job training and crime reduction. Soaring prices and reduced income led to priority dilemmas and stark choices: prevention vs. post-diagnostic intervention, food vs. medicine, the possibility of future AIDS vs. the reality of immediate needs and a diminished ability to afford housing, food and clothing.

All four sites that the RARE investigation focused upon are part of this vast zone of inner-city poverty. The following are their demographic profiles:

Only Site 1 showed an increase in population between 1999 and 2000. The other three sites have experienced a reduction in population. As development and gentrification are spreading across the District, families are being displaced. Many are being relocated to suburban areas of bordering states. Site 1 is located in the ward with the largest white population (53%) and Latino population (7%). Site 4 is located in the ward with the largest African American population (90%), followed by Sites 3 and 2 respectively. Table 1 provides a comparison of the four sites, related to population, poverty, unemployment, family income and crime (www.dcagenda.org).

Table 7.1: Site Comparisons

	Site 1	Site2	Site3	Site 4
Population 1990	66,103	77,942	83,084	83,176
Population 2000	69,349	74,937	71,503	70,899
Change (%) Pop.	4.9	-3.9	-13.9	-14.8
Poverty Rate (%) 1990	18.1	8.2	15.2	27.4
Poverty Rate (%) 2000	18.7	12.1	20.0	36.0
Children in Poverty (%) 1990	21.8	9.0	10.1	38.0
Children in Poverty (%) 2000	25.2	16.4	28.0	47.1
Unemployment Rate (%) 1990	4.8	6.2	9.2	13.2
Unemployment Rate (%) 2000	8.2	6.6	15.2	22.0
% Persons 16-19 Employ/in School 1990	95.0	87.3	88.1	77.0
% Persons 16-19 Employ/in School 2000	96.7	84.8	90.7	79.1
Average Family Income, 1999	130,571	81,416	54,507	35,221
% Change in Av. Family Inc. 1989-99	17.7	6.0	1.9	-4.9
% HHs Below 200% Poverty 1990	30.7	20.7	31.9	48.9
% Violent Crimes 1998	16.8	11.8	18.1	21.4
% Violent Crimes 1999	14.5	10.5	16.8	18.9
% Violent Crimes 2000	14.6	10.8	16.9	19.8
% Property Crimes 1998	124.5	44.5	55.4	34.9
% Property Crimes 1999	102.7	37.8	48.8	30.6
% Property Crimes 2000	103.8	37.1	48.6	29.9

Source: www.dcagenda.org/pages/nis/comparisontables/comparisontables.htm

All four wards increased in their levels of poverty. Site 4 is located in the ward with the consistently highest levels of poverty. Site 4 also had the highest incidence of children in poverty in 1990, which increased by almost 10% by 2000. Site 2 levels of overall poverty increased slightly, but the percentage of children in poverty decreased from 1980 to 1990, but increased again by 2000. Site 3 experienced a reduction in the percentage of poverty in 1990 from 18.1 to 15.2, but this increased again by 2000 to 20.0. However, this ward experienced a nearly 30% increase in children in poverty by 2000. These increases can be attributed in part to the change in welfare laws and downturn in the economy.

Site 1 had the largest number of individuals with four-plus years of college (52%); Site 4 had the lowest (8%). Site 1 had the lowest unemployment rate (6.8%); Site 4 had the highest (17%). As might be expected, Site 4, given its high percentage of poverty, had the highest unemployment rates across three decades as well as the lowest number of people between ages sixteen to nineteen employed or in school. Site 1 had the highest percentage. The disparity in income across the wards is readily evident. Again, Site 4 is in the ward with the lowest level of average income and highest number of households below 200% poverty in 1990.

Violent crimes were highest in the poorest ward, but property crimes were highest in the wealthiest ward. Site 4 had the highest levels of violent crimes for all three years reported, followed by Sites 3, 1 and 2. However, Site 1 experienced the highest levels of property crimes that may be directly related to its wealthier and more stable social and economic circumstances.

D.C., RARE Method

Study Objectives

The purposes of the District project were to identify and describe specific behaviors engaged in by persons within particular communities, which put them at extreme risk for contracting and spreading HIV/AIDS. Its aims were to assess and describe dynamics of the local epidemic in the four targeted communities. The goal was to explain such activities in order to develop effective, specifically targeted interventions.

The following questions were probed: Where are neighborhood hot spots of risky behaviors and activities associated with HIV/AIDS? What behaviors and activities take place? Who is participating in the behaviors and activities? When do the behaviors and activities take place? Why are the behaviors and activities occurring? How do behaviors and activities occur? What might prevent or decrease previously identified behaviors and activities from happening?

What Was Done

The District's RARE project took place between October 2000 and January, 2001. Four field teams, each comprised of three persons, were assembled to conduct geo-mapping, ethnographic observations, brief street-intercepts, informal interviews, in-depth individual interviews and focus groups. Each field team was responsible for collecting, recording and interpreting data for its assigned site. Members were selected by the D.C. Department of Health's Administration on HIV/AIDS (AHA), based on their familiarity with HIV/AIDS issues and District neighborhoods. Interviews were held with community leaders, drug dealers, sex workers, men who have sex with men, transgenders, drug addicts, people living with HIV/AIDS and other residents. Five police ride-alongs were also undertaken. The two ethnographers maintained ongoing communication with AHA's coordinator, who attended each weekly training and data reporting meeting, and provided logistical and technical assistance.

Teams observed their areas over a 24-hour period to determine the times of greatest risk activity and periods of outreach, if any. Geo-mapping provided a picture of where and when the at-risk activities took place in the community. Cultural experts had the in-depth knowledge needed to achieve a deeper understanding of the beliefs and values held by people who are engaging in risky behaviors. Service providers supplied information on services available in the target area, as well as insights into the beliefs and values of the people who practice risky behavior. Direct observation and geo-mapping continued throughout the project. The teams completed two-hundred seventy-four hours of observation, sixty-five informal interviews/street intercepts, twenty-five cultural expert interviews, eighteen focus groups, and five police ride-alongs.

In November, the ethnographers prepared and presented a report based on the findings of the field teams to the local health department for discussion and clarification. Based on the local health department's assessment, in December, a revised report was then presented by the ethnographers to the advisory group for its consideration, critique and recommendations. Based on revisions by the health department and recommendations from the advisory group, a final report by local health officials was to be submitted to the mayor by February 2001 for consideration and action steps. This report has not yet been submitted. Such inaction reinforces residents' cynicism. As one person put it: "We are tired of surveys and the government does nothing in reality. In practice, there is no program, only on paper, and nothing really reaches the community. Let them do something for the community instead of making false promises."

Findings

What follows are summations of pertinent results from each site, based on geo-mapping, observations, street intercepts, focus groups, interviews and police ride-alongs.

Site 1: P Street

Description of Neighborhood

The targeted research site is herein referred to as 'P Street NW' and is commonly called P Street or P Street Beach by locals and visitors. The site includes part of Rock Creek Park west and south of the junction of P Street and 22 Street, there are also several nearby establishments, including Soho Cafe, Fireplace and Mr. P's bars, Badlands dance club, and Omega nightclub and bar. These locales are meeting places for gays and others seeking social and sexual interaction. Establishments on P Street, NW, stay open until 4 a.m. Motorized traffic for paid sex takes place on N Street, located next to a soccer field.

Ethnographic data were also collected around N Street, NW, between 22nd Street and Pennsylvania Avenue. Sexual cruising also occurs in this area.

Greater P Street NW is a wooded area with shelter from dense trees and bushes. A river on one side limits access to it. The wooded section where most sexual activity takes place is adjacent to a grassy, sloped area containing an open-air swimming pool and a soccer field used by both gay and straight people for recreational activities. The woods are criss-crossed by a series of dirt paths, which facilitate cruising by the "patron." During the winter, with a loss of leaves there is much less cover for daylight sexual activities, but nighttime darkness provides sufficient cover. One of two bridges over the river is used by patrons to shield their sexual acts underneath.

Specific Findings

Cruising and sex between gay men take place in wooded areas. Used condoms, lubricants and toilet paper can be readily seen. The surrounding area is used for pick-ups involving men in cars soliciting men who are walking/cruising the streets and vice versa. Some cars have Maryland or Virginia license plates. Straight and gay Latino, African American and white patrons use the site for sexual pick-ups and activity.

The peak hours of greatest sexual activity are between 11 p.m. and 4 a.m., when bars and clubs close, and while people are under the influence of drugs such as ecstasy, marijuana, cocaine and alcohol. There is also risk from sharing infected needles. Partying, drinking and drugging sometime continue in secret houses called chiviadas where unprotected sex is sold by transvestites and bought by self-identified straight men.

No HIV/AIDS prevention information is to be found, even in cafés that are meeting places for gays, nor were any representatives from any HIV/AIDS outreach organizations. Community resources are not mobilized to inform and protect. Some persons do not know where to locate HIV/AIDS services.

Some respondents have had an HIV test, but have not returned to get their results because, "they are not ready nor do they have all the information to deal with the thought of living with HIV." Others have not been re-tested. Many HIV-positive persons do not inform their partner(s) of their sero-status for fear of being rejected.

Condoms are not used consistently because they cause loss of erection and decreased sensitivity. However, one person reported: "It is very difficult to train people in the use of condoms when they are adults; you have to start when they are children."

Among Latinos, misconceptions and religious and social prejudices towards condom use increase the risk of infection. According to one person: "We need to teach our children that an infected person is not condemned nor is a man who has sex with another man." Because consensual sex with men is repressed in Latin America, Latinos who frequent cruising and sex areas may be seduced by the openness and seeming freedom of participating in unprotected oral and anal sex. Large sectors of Latino immigrants are unable to utilize English-only HIV/AIDS information.

HIV/AIDS appears not to be seriously regarded as a life-threatening disease and/or the risks associated with unprotected sex may outweigh the benefits of liberated and pleasurable sexuality. As one person said: "I put myself at risk for pleasure and because I don't have a regular partner."

Risky behaviors are engaged in for several major reasons, including:

- Fewer gay people appear to be dying from HIV/AIDS.
- There is scant condom distribution at targeted sites at selected times, to reduce risk-taking behavior by particular risk categories.
- There is minimum discussion about the social, cultural and medical contexts of HIV/AIDS. HIV/AIDS is no longer perceived as a gay disease.
- Frank discussions of these and related reasons for unprotected sex are not openly or systematically identified and discussed in health and social forums.
- Unsafe, anonymous and unprotected sex takes place in well-known cruising areas during warm weather. In the winter, sexual pursuits occur in bars and clubs, and unprotected sex acts often take place in cars and houses. These activities require specific targeting for health materials and condoms.
- Oral sex is not viewed as a risk.

Community resources for informing and caring for HIV/AIDS are not coordinated. Fragmented approaches exist. Comprehensively planned efforts are needed to identify, incorporate and mobilize neighborhood residents, visitors and business proprietors, especially clubs and bars. In the view of one respondent: "Education, education, education is the key to avoiding the spread of HIV/AIDS."

Site 2: Petworth

Description of Neighborhood

Located in Ward 4, the boundaries of the northwest Petworth research site are: Webster Street on the north, Seventh Street and New Hampshire Avenue to the east, Girard Street on the south, and 14th Street on the west. It is primarily a residential neighborhood of multi-ethnic groups and nationalities, numerous small businesses, row homes, and apartment buildings. A library, churches, and public and private schools are located there. Abandoned and unoccupied buildings are scattered throughout the community.

The Petworth field team concentrated its efforts within the immediate geographical radius of the Fourth Metropolitan Police District of Columbia headquarters located on Georgia Avenue and Peabody Street, NW. This area of Georgia Avenue is a wide and extensive commercial strip of barbershops, beauty parlors, liquor stores, grocery markets, repair shops, clothing stores, meat stores, `girlie' bars, strip clubs, taverns, and other `Mom and Pop' enterprises. It has major bus routes for transporting folks to and from Silver Spring, Maryland, as well as from lower and upper northwest, to various parts of the District, via transfers to other buses and connections to Metro train lines.

Most residents are African American. Central American, Caribbean and African immigrants also live in and frequent the area as reflected in the stores and shops which sell reggae music, and West Indian and Central American baked goods and foods. The Latino population is increasing as residents and clientele although they are fewer in number. Most are from El Salvador, Honduras and Guatemala. Some residents commute between the District and Silver Spring and Hyattsville, Maryland. The few persons of Asian heritage are primarily store owners. At the time of this project, most whites in the area appeared to be police officers.

The reigning posters along Georgia Avenue are huge, colorful weekly announcements of hip-hop and rap concerts. They are tacked on trees and utility poles, tied to street lamps and glued on walls. Other fliers dramatically advertise political events or declare support for some cause. There are no HIV/AIDS posters.

Prevention and outreach workers lack experience and familiarity with Latino, Caribbean and African residents. Potential recipients of HIV/AIDS prevention and treatment are not comfortable or willing to freely discuss and learn about the disease or to seek supportive health services. Residents express concerns about the disease's impact and the need to develop more culturally inclusive educational HIV/AIDS programs. They are extremely dissatisfied with being by-passed or culturally ignored. Most risk is linked to use of dirty needles, anal and oral sex for crack or money, impairment because of alcohol and other drug use, and barriers to utilization of services. Particularly strong barriers are norms that preclude discussion of 'private' or 'sexual' matters outside of the family.

Specific Findings

Geo-mapping, field observations, focus groups, in-depth individual interviews, street intercepts and a police ride-along led to the following findings for Petworth. Petworth's residents have serious unmet needs that confine their ability and willingness to reduce risky behaviors and immediately respond to HIV/AIDS outreach efforts. Among the commonly identified unmet needs are: access to affordable apartments, unawareness about how, where, and when to access social services, legal aid, access to benefits, acquisition of appropriate HIV/AIDS education, help in obtaining non-HIV/AIDS medication, fiscal support, job training, employment and child care.

Major hot spots for risky behaviors of injecting drug use and unprotected sex are: crack houses on Kennedy Street, crack dealing and use on Longfellow Street, sex work and trading along Georgia Avenue and around Randolph Street between Eighth and Fourteenth Street, and heroin selling and use on Georgia Avenue's west side between Morton Street and New Hampshire Avenue. Other drug dealing and use sites include Hamilton, Madison, Oak, Shepherd, Taylor and Webster Streets.

Heroin users in Petworth are at risk for AIDS because of their tendency to share dirty needles and to engage in unprotected commercial sex for money. Vulnerability is increased during the first of the month when people receive entitlement checks, and between 6–9 a.m. when they are trying to get a high, which may last the remainder of the day. Crack cocaine users are at risk because of their compulsive activities designed to trade unprotected sexual acts for crack or participate in sexual activity for money. They are vulnerable throughout the day, but especially when their high moderates. For crack and heroin users, high-risk activities frequently take place in parks, alleys, hallways and apartments. Non-addicted prostitutes, whose 'services' are sold or traded without protection, are at risk for both contracting and spreading AIDS.

Some interviewees labeled users as "crack-heads" and "dope fiends" who should be targeted by police and health officials for isolation and removal from the community. Others deemed them sick people desperately in need of help. In both cases, participants regarded Petworth as a community that has historically and detrimentally lacked vital services.

Targeting socially natural meeting places may be helpful, e.g., gas stations, laundromats, stores, churches, restaurants and related neighborhood locales with informative and linguistically appropriate posters, fliers, pamphlets and brochures. Respondents recommended providing comprehensive HIV/AIDS services linked to helping residents obtain other social and medical services. Although interviewees identified particular hot spots and times for HIV/AIDS, they asserted that risky unprotected sex, and heroin and crack use take place "all year, wherever there are people, anyplace" like clubs and parties. Hence people must be targeted where they socially interact.

There are three distinct categories of "illicit" drug users in Petworth: heroin users in their thirties, forties and fifties; crack cocaine users, generally in their thirties; and marijuana users, typically in their twenties and adolescence. Heroin is generally sold in the mornings. Dealers range from thirteen to forty-four years of age. A heroin high may lasts all day. Users purchase heroin in the morning, get high soon after, and the high lasts until the next day. The cycle is then repeated. These heroin users are "an older crowd," generally in their thirties and older.

The west side of Georgia Avenue is an intense hot spot for heroin purchases. Users are sometimes "standing up asleep and falling asleep—in mid-air." Because a heroin high is longer lasting than crack, "heroin addicts are generally off the street once they get it and get high."

The chemical effects of the two drugs create different social results. Because heroin users in Petworth are typically high in some apartment or house, they usually do not come out throughout the day to sell or purchase sex. Their longer lasting high creates a sedated, mellow, on-going sensation. On the other hand, crack's sensations are shorter and more intense. Users crave greater amounts and want the drug more frequently. Crack users keep coming back frequently to buy or use sex to trade or earn money for more crack. "Crack addicts come and go. Once the high is gone, they will be off gigging for more," i.e., soliciting their bodies for drugs or money to purchase drugs. They are typically in their twenties and thirties.

Local prostitution is linked to cocaine and heroin use, especially crack. Commercial sex workers solicit from early morning and throughout the day. They charge $100 to $200.

Although, commercial sex activity is perhaps more noticeable at night, the busiest time for heroin related prostitution is 6–8 a.m. Users tend to be out seeking the drug or money for the drug most intensely during this period. Prostitution is more prevalent along the commercial and transportation routes of Georgia Avenue than it is along less traveled blocks. Since there is greater car and pedestrian traffic along Georgia Avenue, the sex trade is better for users. Moreover, police tend to patrol less traveled routes. Hence, the prostitutes run into less static. "Because of traffic, it is easy to solicit for sex and to panhandle for money along Georgia Avenue."

On one hot spot, at Eighth and Longfellow Streets, both residential streets, women stand on the corner soliciting sex. Kennedy Street is also a main circuit for prostitutes. "A john picks them up in his car to get drugs, get high, get sex; and then he drops them back off on Kennedy Street." Such activity helps to spread AIDS. A principal hot spot for crack dealing is Eighth and Kennedy Streets, NW. The one hundred block of Kennedy Street is also a site for heroin use. Heroin users have been seen "standing up and high" in that area.

Major sites for heroin dealing and use are 14th Street and Randolph Street, NW, and 14th Street and Monroe Street, NW. Here, male and female heroin users congregate. However, "heroin users generally don't mix with crack users." These two types of users do not hang out together because their chemical and social needs are different. However, alcohol drinkers are mixed in with heroin users. Heroin users may also be found in a park at 14th and Oak Streets. "Once they get their hit, users will sleep in the park after using heroin, and will be up before the sun comes up." Alcohol use is prevalent, as is poly-drug use, especially at clubs and dances. Impaired judgment while inebriated increases the risk of infection from unprotected, casual sex.

Although heroin and crack users tend to get high at different times and in different ways, with distinct social behaviors, there are certain times of the month when general drug use, drug selling and prostitution are higher. Drug dealers, users and commercial sex workers are most intense on the first of the month. They chase checks. When people's entitlement and other checks arrive, so do the dealers and prostitutes. "All types of users and ladies of the night are active between 3 a.m. and 9 a.m. for the first day's checks. When checks come in, that brings all the addicts out. Prostitution picks up. It's a means of support. By the second and third of the month, the users' checks are spent. Then they are out selling their bodies." This cycle is repeated monthly.

Drug dealing is affected by seasonal weather. When the temperature is warm, there are more people hanging out, buying and selling drugs, soliciting sex, and using drugs.

Commercial sex activity is related to drugs of choice. Prostitutes addicted to heroin tend to be older, in their thirties and up to fifty-five years of age. One location for their sex work is Eighth and Kennedy Streets, NW. They are not always alert. They are also not particularly afraid of or concerned with HIV/AIDS transmission. "Some are asleep in cars with their engines running."

Prostitutes addicted to crack are younger than heroin-using women. They range from twenty-five years of age and up. These sex workers and their crack-using customers, as well as crack users generally are fearful of contracting HIV/AIDS. "The younger generation is more afraid of AIDS."

Heroin is primarily injected. Many users tend to carry spoons for snorting. Crack users carry a pipe or piping device for use. Crack and heroin users pose related, yet different health risks and criminal justice issues. Crime is more crack-related. Crack addiction is intense, and the high does not last long. Hence, dependency and craving lead to desperation. "Crack users will do pretty much anything to get crack." Conversely, heroin use is not particularly linked to violent or property criminal offenses. Heroin addicts tend to panhandle and solicit sex, rather than assault, burglarize or steal. After obtaining their heroin, users get high and generally do not need to keep returning for continued injections. They may also just hang around for hours panhandling, especially in the early morning around 6 a.m. Yet these heroin users do not seem to be as desperate as crack users.

On the 600 rear block of Kennedy Street near Longfellow Street, one side of which opens into an alley with a large parking lot next to an apartment building, unprotected sex for drugs and money between men and women sometimes takes place there in vans between 8 p.m. and 2 a.m. Also people deal and use drugs in the alley. Cars circle the blocks looking for users. Most have District license plates. Many have Maryland plates. A few Pennsylvania temporary tags can be seen. Taxis also drop off customers for drugs and sex.

People whose behaviors place them at risk from contracting AIDS cannot be easily stereotyped. Sometimes a female heroin or crack user who is coming down from her high may approach a dealer at a vulnerable time for more ingestion. According to one respondent:

> That's when they are at risk for getting and spreading AIDS. She could be someone's wife. She looks fresh. That's one he wouldn't mind being with. That's where sex for drugs comes in.

On one block is a "real hot store"—a site for heroin dealing. The owner was previously locked up for selling illegal drug paraphernalia. Steady streams of customers, mainly Black, although occasionally white and Latino, go in and out of the market. They never leave with groceries. No evident packages are carried out of the store. Some customers are well dressed. Many have pagers. Some ride by in cars with Virginia tags, park several blocks away, walk to the market, and leave seemingly empty-handed.

A few local laundromats are operated by Latinos and service both blacks and Latinos. One, on Georgia Avenue, is a site of protected and unprotected sexual intercourse among Latino teenagers. Some youth engage in anal and oral sex, believing such acts do not constitute sexual intercourse or loss of one's virginity.

Persons noted that Petworth is not the target of preventive measures or effective efforts to curtail heroin and crack use and commercial sex. Specific messages and handouts related to HIV/AIDS are not provided. Community-based organizations are required to work extensively to gain confidence and trust from residents. The absence of culturally based HIV/AIDS services has created or reinforced a sense of neglect and unconcern about HIV/AIDS.

Residents lack specific knowledge about eligibility requirements, procedures and activities for programs. Others reflected suspicion and deemed the spread of HIV/AIDS to be a government plot which could be stopped. Even so, they also advocated for more services.

Given Petworth's multicultural composition, but non-culturally specific programs, service utilization is low. Materials tend not to be printed in French, Haitian Creole, Jamaican Patois, Spanish dialects, Amharic or other languages spoken and read by Ethiopians and other African immigrants. Residents reported a need for sensitivity training by program administrators. Needle exchange programs were requested. Injecting drug use is viewed as serious risk behavior.

Misconceptions affect risk and propel people to take chances. Some individuals presume that protected sex is only necessary if their partner's physical appearance is sickly.

Site 3: Trinidad

Description of Neighborhood

Trinidad, located in Ward 5, is bounded by West Virginia Avenue, Mount Olivet Road, Bladensburg Road, and Florida Avenue, NE. The area is primarily an African American residential area consisting of row houses and apartment buildings, many of which are Section 8 housing. The community has numerous 'Mom and Pop' stores and liquor stores in and around the community. A local market has outside pay phones that constantly have young men standing around them. Each street appears to have some abandoned buildings, some of which serve as crack houses. Holbrook Terrace has an abundance of boarded-up buildings.

This community was at one time referred to as "Little Vietnam" because of the high number of homicides. Signs of gentrification are seen sporadically throughout the community. One resident noted that Trinidad was considered by some to be part of Capitol Hill. The community is afflicted with three basic "blights": drug dealers, abandoned buildings and an inundation of trash, especially in the alleys.

Much of the community consists of grandparents who are raising their grandchildren. The mothers and fathers are frequently lost to jail, drugs, and migration to Prince George's County, Maryland.

Young girls are vulnerable to unprotected oral, anal and vaginal sex because of peer pressure, seduction by older men and misconceptions about how HIV/AIDS is contracted. Sex workers are usually crack addicts who exchange sex for drugs or money and are willing to have unprotected sex in order to get what they need to feed their habits. The need for drugs is so strong in addicts that some parents prostitute their young children to drug dealers in exchange for drugs or money. Although some services exist, lack of public transportation and/or the financial means to use it are barriers for many. No posters or outreach workers were seen in the community throughout the period of the project. However, HIV/AIDS outreach—condom distribution and HIV testing—was reported to be done periodically by an unidentified group.

Specific Findings

Drug dealers and panhandlers, who consist of both alcoholics and drug users, are usually found in the vicinity of the liquor outlets. Most of the buyers are not from Maryland, West Virginia or Virginia. These buyers prefer to come to the District as the laws are much more lax and, if caught, they are more likely to be charged with a misdemeanor, rather than a felony.

"Drug Boys" are easily identified as they are usually gathered in groups on street corners or in front of houses. They seldom walk the streets alone. If a police car approaches, the group scatters or if they are standing in front of a house, they simply step up onto the porch of the house. Police are not allowed to pursue a person on to private property without sufficient cause. In the winter time police easily identify the drug dealers because they sit in parked cars, one man in back and one in front, with the motors running.

Regular customers approach the dealers and the dealers then get in the customers' cars and ride around while completing the deal. The buyers then return the dealers to their cars. New buyers look for gatherings of young men on the street corners, park their cars and then approach the young men.

Sections of Trinidad are known for the type of drugs sold. The 1300 block of Trinidad Street, Neal and Orren Streets, and Montello and Owen Streets are crack and marijuana areas. Levis and 16th Streets is the source of high-quality marijuana. The gas station at Morse and Holbrook is the location for crack and a liquor store on Mt. Olivet is heroin turf. Marijuana comes in packs of 10, 2"x2" bags and crack comes in tiny blue packets about 1/4" square. Drug dealers hide their stashes in the grass, under rocks, in tires, up in trees. Police use dogs to sniff out the drugs. Allies are heavily used and busy drug use areas are littered with discarded drug packets. Police estimated that there were approximately 100 drug dealers in the community. Crack and marijuana dealers are visible throughout the day but sales pick up around rush hour and continue until they reach a peak, around 2:00 a.m.

Ivy City, which is next to Trinidad, is the area recognized as the main heroin strip, but sections of Trinidad are also known as heroin territories. Dealers are out on the streets in the early morning hours after daybreak. Residents in the community confirmed that they had witnessed needle sharing among the heroin users.

One community leader pointed out that young girls hang out around the "Drug Boys" because it makes them feel grown up and important. The drug dealers entice the girls into drugs and sex by offering the "glamorous" life. On a visit to the Center on a weeknight, more than a half dozen dealers were standing on the steps. A dozen young children under the age of twelve were inside participating in recreational activities.

West Virginia Avenue, Mt. Olivet, and the apartment building at Orren and Neal are the sex worker strips, but the women also work in Ivy City which borders Trinidad. Ivy City is also the heavy heroin area in the Trinidad vicinity. The women, mostly crack addicts, work independently, not for pimps. The clientele come from Maryland, Virginia and the District. The women make eye contact with potential customers and gesture with come-ons.

Cars and alleys are the primary locations for sexual encounters, but a few operate out of their apartments. Police identify the areas of sexual activity by the condoms in the alleys. With welfare reform, a number of women have turned to prostitution and drug dealing as alternative sources of income.

Men who have sex with men (MSM) appear to be a very small part of the population. Gays, lesbians and transgenders cruise mainly along Mt. Olivet, West Virginia Avenue and in Ivy City. In the summertime MSMs hang out on the corners of Orren and Neal Streets.

Sex workers are usually crack addicts who exchange sex for drugs or money and are willing to have unprotected sex in order to get what they need to feed their habits.

The need for drugs is so strong in addicts that some parents prostitute their young girls to drug dealers in exchange for drugs or money. One sex worker identified unprotected sex during orgies as placing all participants at risk.

The pressure on young girls to have sex was expressed by one fourteen year old who said, "All kids expect to have sex. You can't avoid it." Another common belief among teenage girls is that a girl will be able to "*get her man*" if she has his baby. This leads to unprotected sex. Just as vulnerable are the welfare women who acquiesce to the desire of their men to have unprotected sex as the men help provide for the household.

Another problem is older men having sex with younger girls. In one case this led to the arrest of a drug dealer who the police had been trying to arrest for a long time but he had been too well protected. An officer was on a call to a home noticed a young girl with a baby in her arms. She looked too young to have a baby. When finished with taking the complaint he asked her if the baby was hers. She said it was. He then asked who the father was. She identified him as the Drug Lord of the neighborhood, an older man in his forties. This led to the man's arrest and conviction on the basis of rape and he is currently in prison. The girl was only fourteen at the time that the Drug Lord enticed her with the promise of money, gifts, and glamour.

No posters or outreach workers were seen in the community throughout the period of the project. A few of the residents referred to seeing posters on buses, at the H Street bus stop and on an abandoned house in the neighborhood.

Several teenage girls and two older males in street intercepts mentioned that two people passed out condoms on a regular basis. The two men also mentioned that a man comes around in a van periodically and does testing for AIDS. He takes a blood test one week and returns the next week with the results. Participants receive food, clothing, toiletries, etc. They could not remember which organization he worked for.

The police and residents interviewed identified two churches active in the community: Holy Land Spiritual Center located in the 1100 block of Montello, and the New Samaritan Church on Florida Avenue. They offer counseling and youth activities. A few police officers are also actively involved in the community.

Residents go to D.C. General Hospital, Howard University Hospital, Providence Hospital or a clinic in the Metropolitan area to receive services. All of these are a considerable distance from the community. One community leader expressed deep concern over the lack of health care facilities in the community for both the young and old people. She described the situation of one elderly woman in the community who had to make two bus transfers in order to get to D.C. General Hospital. "By the time she arrives at the hospital, her blood pressure is elevated and she is a nervous wreck."

Clinics offer HIV/AIDS services. Several respondents could not remember the names of clinics they visited, but had a general sense of their location. AIDS-specific clinics mentioned were Family Medical Center (on Bladensburg Road in Maryland), Max Robinson Clinic, Whitman Walker Clinic, and the Oasis Methadone Drug Treatment Program.

The Oasis Methadone Drug Treatment Facility at 910 Bladensburg Road, NE, has a recording that refers people to "the doctor" when they phone in for information. Oasis does offer HIV Counseling and Testing Services on Thursdays, but no one in the community seemed to be aware of this. Several residents were afraid to go around the clinic as it is located in close proximity to a liquor store and a number of addicts and drug dealers hang out in the vicinity. One person explained that some clients from the methadone program cross the street to the CVS and "terrorize" the place.

Non-profit organizations mentioned that offer HIV/AIDS counseling or information were: Crises Pregnancy Center, Healthy Start, SASHA Bruce, Salvation Army and Whitman Walker. Organizations or businesses that provide basic information and referrals are: the CVS Health Connection/Family Resource Center, Family Practices Medical Services, and the Northeast Community Improvement Corporation.

The CVS Health Connection/Family Resource Center at the corner of Benning and Bladensburg Roads, NE, had only a minimal amount of information on HIV/AIDS in the form of a pamphlet, and when asked for further information people are referred to the D.C. Department of Health.

Site 4: Barry Farms

Description of Neighborhood

Barry Farms is a closed African American residential community located in Ward 8 in the southwest quadrant of the city. It has the highest incidence of heterosexual female and pediatric AIDS cases in Washington. The area is well known for its drug dealing. Barry Farms is composed of three parallel streets, Stevens Road, Eaton Road and Sumner Road, bounded by Wade Street on the northwest, and Firth Sterling on the southeast. Interstate 295 runs parallel to the community on the southern end. Barry Farms does not have any businesses located within the community. The Anacostia Metro Station is located two blocks north of the community. The two-story apartment dwellings are clusters of connected duplexes. The alleys and open areas between buildings are littered with paper and trash.

Martin Luther King (MLK) Avenue and Good Hope have a plethora of liquor stores and 'Mom and Pop' stores (e.g., Martin's Food Store, Serve Quick, and King's Market) that sell wine and beer. The 2400 block of MLK Avenue has five liquor stores. One of the neighborhoods major liquor stores, Big King's Liquor Store is directly across from the Max Robinson Clinic and is open from 9:00 a.m. until 10:00 p.m. Liquor stores/outlets serve as gathering places for drug dealers, drug addicts, MSMs, sex workers, and panhandlers.

Specific Findings

The Recreational Department located on Sumner Road offers tutoring for the young people and has a swimming pool and basketball courts. At one time there were a lot of vocational and educational programs for youth living in Barry Farms. Football, basketball, and baseball teams provided neighborhood kids with after-school activities. The day care center closed, and now, after school, children go to the Spiritual Center located on Stevens Road. This center offers GED classes to drop-outs and a computer class to interested community residents. Residents patronize businesses, medical services, and liquor stores along Martin Luther King Avenue and Good Hope Road. The Max Robinson Clinic, Family Medical and Counseling Services, two medical facilities located on MLK Avenue are available to residents of Barry Farms. Whitman Walker Clinic, Safe Haven, D.C. General Hospital's Phoenix Program, Children's Hospital, Umoja, D.C. Cares, SASHA Bruce, Metropolitan Teen AIDS, HIV Support Groups, HIV Hot Lines, HIV Ministries and St. Elizabeth's Hospital were other places the CRT found were known and used by residents.

The Anacostia Community Health Center, located on W St., SW, does not have HIV/AIDS counseling available at the clinic as a separate program. OB/GYN screenings have uncovered some cases. Adult patients are counseled and then referred out to the Phoenix program at D.C. General Hospital; children are referred to Children's Hospital. The clinic produces monthly newsletters on HIV/AIDS. On the adult side of the clinic a bulletin board is dedicated to HIV/AIDS.

The side effects of the crack epidemic are becoming painfully evident in the local elementary school, Vern Elementary. "The crack babies are totally out of control and exhibit violent behavior. Teachers are having a very difficult time controlling the kids. But it isn't really the kids' fault, because they got damaged by the crack that passed to them from their mothers." Women are not always aware of how drugs affect the fetus.

The Southeast Community Collaborative is composed of churches, individuals and community organizations including the Max Robinson Clinic. This organization attempts to expose the children and adults to the broader community and help residents to understand the relationship between their community and the Metropolitan area. Many people never leave the small enclave of their local community. One community leader who works with the organization complained that, "It is extremely difficult to get the parents involved. Unless you are giving something away or offering food they won't come to an activity." Children and adults are taken on fieldtrips in order to try and broaden their views of life. The need for this type of activity was evident on a recent field trip to Georgetown when the kids thought they were in Maryland. It was their first trip outside of Barry Farms.

The Collaborative and police provide the staff at the Recreational Center with free tickets to basketball games and other activities when possible. Two churches active in the community that offer programs for children are Matthew's Memorial and Campbell AME. Young women, bisexual males, injecting drug users, sex workers, victims of domestic violence and people under the influence of drugs/alcohol are at risk. Sex, drugs and high risk-behavior are inextricably intertwined. Young women who knowingly take drugs or drink alcohol lose their inhibitions and judgment, resulting in unprotected sex. Sex workers and the customers they serve, many of whom come from neighboring states, risk their lives when they have unprotected sex for more money. Persons who share dirty needles are also at risk.

Bisexual males who engage in unprotected anal, oral and/or vaginal sex are conduits for the spread of AIDS between the gay and heterosexual populations. "Gold digging" increases the risk of HIV/AIDS infection for all involved – this is a practice in which a woman caters to a select group of men for support (usually older pensioners). Returning ex-offenders are another potential vector for spreading the disease. Approximately 2,000 men return to the District each year from prison.

Recommendations

The following are recommendations drawn from the research to reduce the spread of HIV/AIDS in the District:

For Injectors

> Recommendation 1: Teams need to be trained to provide outreach and services on a 24-hour basis, not 9 a.m. to 4 p.m.

A major finding by the field teams was the lack of outreach in the communities during the peak times when the most at-risk behavior takes place. For example, heroin users are most at risk in the early hours before sunrise. Crack users are more at risk in the late-night and early-morning hours. Prostitutes are more at risk the later in the night it becomes because of the need to get money and their willingness to do what it takes to get it.

> Recommendation 2: Supply AIDS kits, needle sterilizing packets, condom machines and literature to local businesses and neighborhood meeting places, e.g., barber shops, beauty salons, grocery stores and liquor stores.

This was a recurrent request by community residents in all four sites. They stressed that the availability of resources is an important step in combating the disease's spread.

Access to Services

> Recommendation 3: Bring mobile health vans to communities on a regular basis that offer "general health care services," in addition to testing, counseling and referrals for HIV/AIDS services.

Sending mobile vans into communities for the purpose of testing and counseling was met with a marked lack of enthusiasm. Residents pointed out that the stigma attached to the illness prevented many people from being tested in programs that targeted only HIV/AIDS. As many residents have multiple health concerns, the offering of general health services could bring better health care management to communities in general, while also focusing on HIV/AIDS prevention and treatment.

> Recommendation 4: Provide free transportation to hospitals and clinics that offer HIV/AIDS testing and treatment services.

The levels of poverty in communities in the District place transportation to medical facilities that offer testing and services beyond the financial capability of many families. Providing transportation would allow individuals to access services without the stigma of being seen entering a mobile van designated for HIV/AIDS work.

Cultural and Health

> Recommendation 5: The active involvement and representation of Latino, African and Caribbean organizations on planning councils and programs related to family care and HIV/AIDS prevention, treatment and care are essential for programmatic success.

This was strongly emphasized by residents. Work in Site 2 brought into sharp focus the lack of services and resources for Latino, African and Caribbean communities.

> Recommendation 6: Provide literature and personnel versed in the languages and cultures of the sites' various ethnic groups.

Health care, prevention, utilization, intervention and treatment rely on culturally competent services and linguistically appropriate and relevant materials.

> Recommendation 7: Provide culturally and linguistically relevant pre- and post-test counseling and financial incentives for persons to be tested and return for their results.

This approach may help increase the numbers of people who return for their HIV test results.

> Recommendation 8: Mandatory testing of customers of commercial sex workers should be implemented.

Many customers come from the bordering states of Virginia and Maryland, as well as West Virginia and Pennsylvania. Requiring testing of customers was recommended by many participants to help prevent HIV transmission to unsuspecting spouses or significant others.

> Recommendation 9: As an aspect of educational programs, include student visits to hospitals, nursing homes and hospice centers where they can meet with AIDS patients.

First-hand experience with persons with HIV/AIDS may help dispel false ideas and perceptions as to the causes of the disease and its impact on individual lives. Students could conduct HIV/AIDS research or service learning projects. One specific project mentioned was to have students construct memorial trees in their schools to schoolmates and neighborhood children who have died from HIV/AIDS.

> Recommendation 10: Develop alliances between police and health care workers to identify and target times and locations where and when risky activities take place and where services are most needed.

According to residents, an underutilized source in the fight against the spread of HIV/AIDS is the police force. This is particularly important in light of the fact that these areas where risky behaviors take place do not remain static.

> Recommendation 11: HIV/AIDS-reduction policies must be formulated, conducted and assessed within a broader framework of sustainable community development that enhances the structural living conditions of marginalized residents.

Respondents and field observations noted that HIV/AIDS in the District appears to be most prevalent in neighborhoods and among people who suffer unequal access to health care and other institutional requirements for a healthy life.

Lessons Learned: Implications for Policy Changes

Project Inception

The Washington, D.C., RARE project did not allow for sufficient time between the project's notification and inception. The ethnographers had less than a week's notice. Ethnographers would benefit from a briefing by the Health Department beforehand on departmental initiatives, policies, programs and resources. The local health officials and advisory committee members should be provided with a session in the basics of ethnographic work (re: philosophy, purpose, rationale, methods, process, analysis and assessment) to reduce the possibility of later misunderstandings concerning the process, the results and recommendations. For example, at one point, a health official was asked to provide a list of the services available in a particular community; the sarcastic response was, "Isn't that what the CRTs [Crisis Response Teams] are supposed to be finding out?" Development and use of academically appropriate modules that specify and clarify administrative and ethnographic tasks such as recording field observations, note-taking and conducting focus groups should be done in the project's early stages.

Logistics, Roles, Timetables

The logistics, field responsibilities, end products and timetables for completion of activities need to be clearly spelled out at the beginning of the project. It is particularly important to clarify project roles, objectives and relationships between federal health officials, District health officials, the evaluator and ethnographers. Gray areas of responsibility lead to lost time and undermine team-building efforts. This became particularly evident in the end-stages of the project when the draft of the final report was being prepared and presented.

Team Selection

Another caution is warranted in the area of selection of field team members. In the District, the field teams were selected prior to the ethnographers coming onto the project. Participating in the selection process can avoid later problems with team members who do not have the minimum skills required to do the tasks. Knowledge of a community or personal experience is insufficient qualification for this project. Commitment and time are primary characteristics, as well as an individual's ability to enter any neighborhood and be flexible with the insider and outsider roles. Ethnographers are more aware of what is needed and can explain better what is expected.

Training

Training is critical to the success of the project. Prior to the teams entering the field, they received two days of what normally was a three-day training program. Ongoing training was provided at weekly meetings. Training was designed to reinforce the in-field activities that team members were doing at the time. A major problem for field team members was differentiating between data collection and service. To help resolve this issue, members distributed condoms in their sites while doing their geo-mapping. They also were told to avoid making promises of services after the research ended, as it was unclear what was going to happen with the report and what action would be taken on the recommendations. The District's project would have been aided by greater logistical contractor technical assistance in the form of training to help resolve participants' confusion between their research and outreach roles.

Field Team Responsibilities

How team members spent their time and the number of hours spent on a given activity became a problem. Clearly specifying the average number of hours per week each field team member can work for the project's duration is critical. An alternative to hourly wages is to link field team payments to tasks and deliverables of team members, which would be reviewed by ethnographers. Product-based payments, rather than hourly wages, would improve the quality of research, data collection, analysis and reports.

Meetings

Weekly team meetings were held throughout the project. The Health Department liaison participated in all of the meetings, and occasionally a member of the advisory committee attended the meetings. On several occasions, the ethnographers met with each team separately from the weekly meeting to work on specific issues or to update members. It would be helpful for ethnographers to hold bi-monthly meetings/training sessions for separate teams, in addition to the collective weekly team training. This would allow the ethnographers to address the individual needs of team members, as each team member comes with a different level of technical abilities and skills.

Involvement of the advisory committee throughout the process should be encouraged. The more aware committee members are of the process, the more meaningful the report and recommendations will be. The evaluator attended meetings half-way through the project and at the end of the project. No feedback was given. Direct feedback at each stage would enrich the process.

Final Report

As the draft of the final report was being prepared, it became evident that some informational or analytical gaps existed in the data collection. Additional time should be allotted at the beginning of a project to allow for these gaps to be addressed, prior to submission of the final report. Time should also be scheduled for each field team member and site team to review and comment on the ethnographer's final draft reports to the District health officials and advisory committee.

It is important to clarify roles and responsibilities in the editing process after submission of the ethnographers' final draft reports. Input by the ethnographers is important at all stages to guarantee the integrity of the data reported and recommendations made. A set time for feedback from the advisory committee on the final draft should be set and followed. In the case of the District, health officials distributed the final report to the advisory committee for comment, but waited until they heard back from everyone. This has contributed to the long delay in submission. The specific deadline for submission of the final report to the mayor for action should be designated at the beginning of the project and then honored.

Summary

In theory, RARE is based on scientific methodology, community participation and collaborative technical assistance. It is a relatively rapid process of initiation, conceptualization, endorsement, data collection, findings, recommendations and implementation. Data are collected in specific neighborhoods at different time periods through geo/community mapping, participant observation, personal interviews, street intercepts, focus groups and police ride-alongs. The methodology is fairly simple in theory and straightforward in application. The research is mainly ethnographic, although quantitative data are also collected. Those who know and feel comfortable in the community and its culture are the best people to conduct the fieldwork. Perspectives from insiders and outsiders are obtained. To the extent that they are heard and utilized as one component of policy planning, the spread of HIV/AIDS will no longer be seemingly relentless.

As envisioned, RARE is a form of community-based research which can provide data useful for program planning and evaluation. It can assist quantitative survey planning and interpretation of statistical data. RARE is a tool for informing community participation and decision-making in research, program planning, implementation and evaluation.

RARE projects need to be standardized without losing their creativity and community-based focus. Scientists, policy makers and community researchers also need to evaluate the methodology. Developing and standardizing methods of rapid research and technical assistance will expand the field and provide greater credibility, validity and reliability. RARE has much potential for helping communities and public officials to develop, implement and evaluate new approaches that are not dismissive, disruptive or threatening to targeted communities.

One of RARE's strengths is that it provides health care providers and policy makers with the perspective of individuals at risk on the causes of and solutions to the spread of HIV/AIDS. A potential problem occurs when suggestions from the community are in conflict with previous findings. For example, residents across sites strongly suggested the need to provide AIDS kits and sterilizing kits in local socializing spots. However, members of AHA and the advisory committee were not very receptive to this recommendation.

It is also important to explore new avenues and partnerships in the fight against AIDS (Quimby and Friedman 2003). This may include overcoming prejudices and stereotypes about potential partners. For example, building partnerships between police and health care workers in an effort to identify hot spots and times of risky behavior met with resistance from some members of the advisory committee who hold a totally negative view of the relationship of police with the community members they serve. However, in the police ride-alongs, it was evident that many police officers work at building good relationships with the residents of communities they serve–including drug dealers, prostitutes and juveniles, as well as families.

Conclusion

In the District, prevention of HIV has been stifled by bureaucracy, lack of community control over the technical assistance process, fragmented health care delivery, and competing issues and concerns of community residents. Despite all the data, findings, analyses, conclusions and recommendations, in the mix is institutional inertia sustained by a political economy that minimally responds to culturally de-centered and economically marginalized people. This has been more than clearly exemplified in the District's RARE effort by the fact that the report has not been forwarded in a timely fashion to the mayor for action. Information and knowledge are hardly power. This lack of follow-through only frustrates community residents in terms of participation in efforts to bring prevention and treatment programs to their communities. Entering three decades of facts, the struggle against HIV and AIDS in the District of Columbia appears to have by-passed those who have been most attacked by the epidemic.

It is a truism (although imperative) to assert that prevention and treatment should be culturally competent and responsive to targeted people. It is also a cliché (yet essential) to note that health care exists within multiple contexts. To be consistently effective, applying RARE theory to grounded conditions in the District requires political structures, social values and economic resources that enable or force people and institutions to deliver life-saving interventions. Without power, such delivery is a rare event.

References

CDC. (2003) *HIV AIDS Surveillance Reports*. 1985–2002. Atlanta: Centers for Disease Control and Prevention.

CDC. (1998) *Trends in the HIV and AIDS Epidemic*. Atlanta: Centers for Disease Control and Prevention.

HHS. (1999) HHS announces three sites for special crisis response teams to battle HIV/AIDS in minority communities. [press release, June]. U.S. Department of Health and Human Services.

HHS. (2000) *Healthy People 2010*. Washington, D.C.: U.S. Department of Health and Human Services.

Manderson, L., Aaby, P. (1992) "An Epidemic in the Field? Rapid Assessment Procedures and Health Research," *Social Science Medicine* 35: 839–850.

Needle, H.R., Trotter, II, R.T., Singer, et al. (2003) "Rapid Assessment of the HIV/AIDS Crisis in Racial and Ethnic Minority Communities: An Approach for Timely Community Interventions," *American Journal of Public Health* 93: 970–979.

Quimby, E., Friedman, S.R. (2003) Dynamics of Black Mobilization against AIDS in New York City. In P. Conrad and V. Leiter (eds.), *Health and Health Care as Social Problems* (pp. 145–159). Lanham, MD: Rowman & Littlefield.

Scrimshaw, S.C.M., Hurtado, E. (1987) *Rapid Assessment Procedures for Nutrition and Primary Health Care: Anthropological Approaches to Improving Programme Effectiveness*. Los Angeles: University of California Latin American Center Publications.

Stimpson, G.V., Fitch, C., Rhodes, T. (eds.)(1998) *The Rapid Assessment and Response Guide on Substance Use and Sexual Risk Behavior*. Geneva: World Health Organization, United Nations Joint Programme on HIV/AIDS.

Trotter, II, R.T., Needle, H.R. (1999) *Crisis Response Teams and Communities Combat HIV/AIDS in Racial and Ethnic Minority Populations: Rapid Assessment, Rapid Response, and Evaluation Field Assessment Training Workbook*. Washington: Office of HIV/AIDS Policy, U.S. Department of Health and Human Services.

Watts, I. and Lewis, R. (2000) *The Administration for HIV/ AIDS and The HIV Prevention Community Planning Committee District of Columbia HIV Prevention Three Year Plan 2000–2002*, District of Columbia: Department of Health.

Online References

AIDS Public Use Data Query Results Washington DC MSA.htm

AIDS Public Use Data Query Results Washington DC MSA Death Status.htm

http://www.dcagenda.org/pages/nis/comparisontables/comparisontables.htm (Sites used within this data base included: Ward_racethnicity.htm; Ward_child_wellbeing.htm; Ward_crime.htm; Ward_family_risk factors.htm; Ward_population.htm)

http://www.cdc.gov/hiv/stats/hasr1302.htm (for information on the District of Columbia)

http://wonder.cdc.gov/AIDSPublic.html

http://dchealth.dc.gov/services/administration_offices/schs/reports.shtm

http://dchealth.dc.gov/services/special_programs/std/reports2001.shtm

Chapter 8

Rapid Assessment in Oakland: HIV, Race, Class, and Bureaucracy

Benjamin P. Bowser
Barbara Hill

Introduction

Ground zero for the rapid spread of HIV in Oakland, California, consists of three interconnected areas. First, there is the old "tenderloin" concentration of single-occupancy hotels, sex parlors, peep shows, and depressed buildings off the downtown. Oakland, like most American cities, went through a period of business and job flight, leaving a depressed downtown. But in recent years, redevelopment has literally created a new downtown and the old depressed space is rapidly disappearing. This older space has a number of congregation sites for men to have homosexual encounters, for injection drug users to buy drugs and shoot-up, and for women and men to engage in commercial sex trading.

The second area of high-risk HIV is in walking distance from the old downtown, across one of two highways that cut across downtown Oakland. It is West Oakland, the oldest, most densely concentrated, and poorest African American community in Oakland. Here there are additional sites where injectors shoot drugs and sex traders work. West Oakland was also the site of "out of control" crack dealing and abuse a decade ago. But now, it is a site for gentrification and is witnessing a rapid influx of Asian and white urban residents who are taking advantage of depressed property values in walking distance from Oakland's downtown and public transportation to San Francisco.

Finally, the third place where HIV infections are epidemic is East Oakland, a large flatland running east for two and one-half miles from the downtown to the city line. African Americans also heavily populate East Oakland, many of whom moved decades ago from West Oakland for better housing and more space. There is also a large Latino community in East Oakland. Both communities have deep pockets of injection drug use, crack use and trafficking, and commercial sex work. The areas of East Oakland closest to the downtown and to the Latino communities in the Fruitvale area are now also coming under increased pressure for redevelopment.

The "tenderloin" surrounding the new downtown and the sites in West and East Oakland account for roughly 90% of the diagnosed AIDS case in the city of Oakland and 70% of all cases in the county, which includes the cities of Berkeley, Hayward, and Alameda. There are other areas with high concentrations of African Americans; but these do not have the same high rates of poverty and unemployment, and of diagnosed AIDS cases and HIV infections. There are many more white residential areas in the city and county with very few AIDS cases. A number of these white communities also have high concentrations of lower and working class residents, as do West and East Oakland. So why are the oldest and most heavily African American communities the sites of the HIV/AIDS epidemic?

Background

The percentage of African Americans in Oakland more than doubled in twenty years, going from less than 2.6% of the population in 1930 to 6.3% by 1944 and 12.4% by 1950. The black population in East Oakland went from 16.2% of the total population in 1940 to 61.5% by 1950. Overcrowding in West Oakland Black households doubled between 1940 and 1950 from 16% of households to 30%. By 1944, Blacks began to move into East Oakland in such large numbers that if the trend continued, it was clear that the City of Oakland would very well became a majority African American city in the foreseeable future (Daniels 1980).

The response to the projected racial demographics for Oakland was swift. Major employers began to leave Oakland. In the first half of the twentieth century, most jobs were in small businesses and government services. By World War II, corporations became the largest and most influential employers. In 1925, 602 establishments in Oakland generated $144 million; 40% ($58 million) was from manufacturing. By 1967, 748 establishments generated $417 million; well over 70% of these revenues were generated by only 243 large establishments. These dominant employers included Kaiser Industries, Owens-Illinois Glass, Montgomery Ward, Transamerica, Sunshine Biscuit Company, Standard Oil of California, Shell Oil, Bank of America, Sears, Roebuck and Company, Mack Trucks, The Dodge Truck Division of Chrysler Motors, Mead Paper Company, The Southern Pacific, Western Pacific, and Santa Fe Railroads, Pacific Telephone and Telegraph, Pacific Gas and Electric, and *The Oakland Tribune* newspaper (Hayes 1972).

Major employers not only began withdrawing jobs, they put brakes on investment for expansion of retail trade in Oakland, as well. Lack of space for plant expansion was the public explanation for disinvestment. Kaiser, Dodge Trucks, Merchant Calculators, Nordstrom Valve, Chevrolet cars, to name a few, all moved plants and offices out of Oakland altogether. The postwar policies of the Oakland Chamber of Commerce de-emphasized Oakland as a site of new manufacturing and retail, and promoted regional development instead. The vehicle for this shift in policy was the Chamber's Metropolitan Oakland Area Program, established in 1935, a year after the 1934 first general strike. The southern reaches of Alameda County became the new site of new investment and jobs. By 1962, Oakland, which had been the heart of manufacturing in the East Bay, was down to 28% of all manufacturing (Hayes 1972).

The flight of good-paying jobs and business from Oakland was further facilitated by post-War federal highway and housing programs. Four developments complemented the flight of labor-intensive jobs from Oakland. First, the Federal highway program expanded existing road access to and from Oakland and opened two new areas to economic and residential development – the 680 Interstate north-south by-pass corridor and the 580 Interstate corridor south and east to Livermore. Improvements to Bay Bridge access routes sent one new highway right through the heart of black West Oakland.

The third development was a federal home loan policy that fueled the development of suburban residential communities along the new highway corridors. African Americans were kept out of these new communities by racial discrimination in mortgage loans and by real estate agents "steering" of black prospective buyers away from new "white" communities (Hunter 1964). Until recently, there were very few African Americans living in San Leandro, Hayward, Fremont, and Castro Valley. This is still the case in Pleasanton, Livermore, Concord, Danville, and Orinda. Finally, labor-intensive industries began to take advantage of cheaper land and easy access along the new federal highway corridors to expand facilities and to build new plants. Meanwhile, many of the industries that remained in Oakland did so because they were obsolete and soon closed.

The separation of well-paying jobs from an increasingly African American, urban, and unionized labor force did not happen by chance. It was a planned and strategic outcome that set the stage for today's deterioration of viable residential communities in both West and East Oakland.

Long-Term Impacts

Between 1959 and 1969, there was a 4.8% decline in the size of the overall labor force in Oakland and a 2% overall decline in population, reflecting disinvestment in manufacturing. The 1969 Oakland civil labor force unemployment rate was 7.9% of 150,987 workers—almost the same rate as in 1959. But from 1959 to 1969, African Americans went from 23% to 34% of Oakland's total population—an 11% increase. But no one told the new immigrants that their economic prospects were in decline. So by 1969, there were at least 8,111 African Americans unemployed. The large unemployed population, primarily in West Oakland, had increased by 30% during the 1960s.

To make matters worse, between 1959 and 1969, West Oakland lost population and housing due to the exhaustion of older buildings, the construction of U.S. Interstate 880, The Bay Area Rapid Transit, and urban renewal. Now the black unemployed alone could entirely populate four census tracts. Their impact and visibility were even greater in 1969 than in 1959. Racial discrimination in jobs and housing did not let up during the 1960s either. African Americans were still confined to employment in dying and moving industries, and to housing in West and East Oakland.

What does increased unemployment mean for communities already suffering high unemployment? First, pockets of poverty that existed prior to 1960 persisted and grew first in West Oakland and then later in East Oakland. Second, the unemployed and their families had to survive on the resources of family, friends, public assistance, and whatever temporary work they could find, much like the unemployed during the Great Depression. Third, income levels in the community went down while the cost of living went up. Fourth, buyers or renters avoided neighborhoods with high unemployment, and people selling property in these neighborhoods found few buyers. Property values sank. Fifth, ratios of renters to owners went up as owners converted single-family homes to multi-unit rentals. With multi-unit rentals came higher population density. Property maintenance went down and blighting accelerated.

The increasing marginalization and impoverishment of the African American working and lower class in Oakland were ignored and, by 1970, blacks were told that they had to make the transition to the new "service economy." But what happened instead is that Mexican immigrants began filling jobs in the new "service" sector of the economy. Why did Latinos end up in these jobs when African Americans were an already existing source of labor? The answer is not that Latinos "took jobs" from African Americans. An explanation closer to reality is that white employers, looking for cheap labor, were reluctant to hire African Americans after a decade of civil rights, protests and race riots, and saw Latinos as a cheap and docile alternative. Service sector employers to this day do not employ African Americans for the very same reason that manufacturers abandoned Oakland—to avoid paying higher wages and benefits to U.S. citizens.

By 1980, Oakland's overall population declined for a second straight decade. Between 1969 and 1979, the overall population decline was 5.8%, from 359,000 to 339,000, more than twice the rate of the prior decade. The primary explanation for the decline was "white flight." A second well-publicized and related change was that Oakland had become nearly a majority black city (46.9%). *The 1980 Census of Population and Housing* showed that tracts where 85% of the population was white declined from 44% in 1969 to 23% by 1979. Predominantly black West Oakland increased in size from 16 tracts to 23, and black East Oakland increased in size from 11 to 25 tracts—more than doubling in size in one decade. Not only were whites displaced by African Americans, African Americans displaced Latinos in several tracts as well.

A tract-by-tract examination reveals how devastating unemployment was. The most densely populated black West Oakland tracts had civilian labor force unemployment rates of 10.4%, 12.6%, and 16.8% [tracts 4010, 4025, and 4016]. But when we compare the adult population with those employed and looking for work between 1950 and 1980, the number of adults not in the labor force increased substantially across all three decades. Who were these people?

The Underclass

In pockets of West and East Oakland, the unemployed were a near-majority of the population and many of the children of the unemployed were themselves unemployed as young adults. These people did not stay invisible. They committed crimes, used and sold drugs, and cost millions in social services as the communities they lived in collapsed as social entities. The discovery of large numbers of unemployed blacks in Oakland did not trigger an examination of its source—the accumulation of thirty years of mounting black economic exclusion from the workforce. What shocked the public was their apparent numbers, the crimes, service costs and their lack of interest in work. Explanation was replaced by blame. Lack of an apparent work ethic became the explanation for their poverty and troubles. Behold, the "black underclass."

Unemployed is defined by the U.S. Department of Labor as those who are looking for work in the legal economy. It does not include those who have stopped looking for work. The black underclass is comprised of people, mostly men, who no longer are looking for work in the legitimate economy after decades of discouragement due to racial discrimination in employment and more recently a preference for lower cost non-citizens. These men and women have been out of gainful employment for so long that they have given up. Still others never acquired meaningful employment. The underclass survives economically by doing illegal "work" which leads to arrests. In turn, employers are reluctant to hire people with jail records, who must receive minimum wages and benefits as U.S. citizens, who lack training and education, and indeed, who often do not have a work ethic.

It is no coincidence that crime rates in West Oakland and the city exploded after 1968. White and black Oakland residents' fear of crime was not irrational. In 1972, Oakland had 28,712 serious crimes that called for police attention—more than double that of the five previous years. By 1977 the number jumped to 42,883 (149% increase) and by 1983 to 44,678 (155%) (Census 1980). The reason why African Americans were associated with this unprecedented crime wave was because the main source of income for the black underclass became heroin trafficking and use.

Heroin and then Crack

When half of the men in one's community are without work, underemployed, and without prospects of a living wage, it is no wonder that so many turn to selling heroin and cultivating users and buyers. Heroin trafficking was no coincidence and its consequences for harm were seen well in advance. The movie "Black Panther" ends with the combined effort of the Oakland Police Department and the Federal Bureau of Investigation to destroy the Panther Party and its leadership who in Oakland actively opposed heroin traffickers. In reality, soon after the Panthers were eliminated, heroin flooded the most impoverished sections of West and East Oakland.

Heroin trafficking and use in West and East Oakland are not based upon recreation or curiosity. They are intrinsically connected to the desperation of large numbers of people living in poverty characterized by long-term high unemployment—the underclass. People shut off from legitimate participation in the economy still have to pay rent, buy food, and have money to survive. Heroin dealing in these communities is first of all about money to survival. Heroin dealing is also about elevating one's social status among peers because of the money earned, and then it is about freedom from menial and degrading work. Heroin dealing is also a form of self-employment and independence.

By 1990, no one could have imagined conditions in West and East Oakland getting worse. But a new drug, crack cocaine, caught parents, police, educators, community organizations, and public health professionals by surprise. Young people who avoided heroin jumped at crack. Crack cocaine was cheap, did not require injection, and was powerfully addictive. Overnight, crack cocaine became the basis of a new alternative economy for marginalized black youth in Oakland. Crack cocaine and the police war on drugs literally brought entire neighborhoods to their knees that were already ravaged by the heroin epidemic. There was a new and even larger wave of muggings, house break-ins, and street crime committed by a new generation of addicts.

The Road to AIDS

Both heroin and crack led to HIV infections and AIDS. It is very likely that HIV initially passed from gay and bisexual injectors to heterosexual injectors through needle sharing. The male and female sex partners of those men were also infected. The result is that HIV became a general epidemic among heroin injectors. Gays, bisexuals, and injectors were the main source of HIV in Oakland prior to 1990. But then crack enflamed the existing epidemic. Young women and men engaged in sexual favors for money to buy crack or to receive crack directly. Injectors who were HIV infected became part of their clientele. The cross-over between heroin injectors and crack users was so complete by 1995, that it became difficult to find injectors who used only heroin. Most also used crack and/or cocaine mixed with their heroin.

It is no coincidence that the increasing numbers of diagnosed AIDS cases and the larger numbers of those who are HIV-positive but have not developed AIDS are from the West and East Oakland communities ravaged by crack. These are the same communities ravaged earlier by heroin. These also are the very same communities with now four decades of accumulated unemployment and poverty.

Rapid Assessment in Oakland, California

The Alameda County Health Officer submitted a letter of intent to conduct a RARE assessment to the Office of HIV/AIDS on December 22, 1998, followed by a formal request for federal assistance on February 9th 1999. The letter pointed out the disproportionate rates of HIV/AIDS among minorities (African Americans) in Alameda County, particularly in the county's largest city, Oakland.

During the three months for which data were collected for the Oakland RARE project, ninety-six new AIDS cases were reported in Alameda County. During this short time period, African Americans accounted for a majority of the cases as shown in table 1.

Table 8.1: Oakland and Alameda County Reported AIDS cases, 5/15–8/15, 2000, by Ethnicity

Race/Ethnicity	Oakland (%)	Alameda County (%)
African Americans	42 (69)	55 (57)
Caucasian Americans	12 (20)	27 (28)
Hispanics	5 (08)	11 (11)
Asian, Native American	2 (03)	3 (03)
Total	61 (100)	96 (100)

Source: Alameda County Department of Public Health

The distribution of risk factors for the reported cases was similar for Oakland and Alameda County. The modes of exposure for the sixty adult/adolescent cases in Oakland are listed in table 2. There were forty-eight AIDS cases diagnosed in males. Men, who cited having sex with other men as a sole risk factor, accounted for a majority of cases (twenty-three cases or 56%). But the most rapidly growing category of exposure was heterosexual contact (twelve cases or 25%).

There were twelve AIDS cases diagnosed in adult/adolescent females in Oakland. Nine of the cases (75%) were attributed to heterosexual contact. The only other mode of exposure listed for females was injection drug use (IDU). In Oakland, the three leading routes of exposure for the total number of cases (male and female) were homosexual contact (45%), heterosexual contact (35%), and IDU (17%). In Alameda County, the proportions attributed to homosexual, heterosexual contact and IDU were 45%, 32%, and 13% respectively (not shown).

Table 8.2: Mode of Exposure for Adult/Adolescent AIDS cases in Oakland Reported from 5/15–8/15, 2000

Exposure	Males (%)	Females (%)	Total (%)
MSM	27 (56)	0 (00)	27 (45)
IDU	7 (15)	3 (25)	10 (17)
MSM & IDU	1 (02)	0 (00)	1 (02)
Heterosexual	12 (25)	9 (75)	21 (35)
Risk not Reported	1 (02)	(00)	1 (02)
Total	48 (100)	12 (00)	60 (100)

Source: Alameda County Department of Public Health

Homosexual contact continues to be the largest exposure category among diagnosed AIDS cases; but cases, based upon injection drug use and heterosexual contact, are increasing rapidly.

The Start of RARE

The RARE oversight committee met on May 1, 2000. They reviewed what was known about the epidemic in Oakland and Alameda County. They then made initial assessments about the scope and focus of the research needed to describe the current status of HIV/AIDS risk-taking in the county and city. This included the known locations where people engage in HIV/AIDS high-risk behaviors, the specific risk groups, the interventions in place, and who conducts those interventions. During this first meeting, the field team was established, consisting of personnel from the Alameda County Public Health Department, and HIV/AIDS outreach and service organizations (H/ASOs).

The field team underwent intensive training from May 2 to 4, conducted by Dr. Robert Trotter in order to learn how to effectively collect qualitative data to characterize the epidemic and risk factors specific to the target areas. Drs. Benjamin Bowser and the late Eleanor Engram conducted subsequent trainings.

The initial observation and mapping fieldwork began May 12, and the first focus group was held June 15. The Oakland RARE programmatic goals were:

- To enhance the community capacity to describe and monitor local risk environments, patterns of behavior and HIV/AIDS epidemic dynamics (Rapid Assessment)
- To use new knowledge to identify and implement interventions to enhance and sustain prevention treatment and care (Rapid Response)
- To examine the impact of the RARE process on the public health system and interventions to vulnerable populations (Rapid Evaluation).

A second working group meeting was held on May 23, introducing the newly trained field team to the oversight committee. The meeting focused on the details of the RARE method and process. The next two months were spent in intensive observations and interviews, area team briefings, training new and additional outreach observers, and interpreting and developing findings.

The RARE Method

In total, over two hundred fifty hours of observation, eight focus groups, fifty-one short interviews, and seven key interviews were performed in the four designated areas: Broadway and Telegraph, Lake Merritt, Fruitvale and the Lower Bottom. Additionally, eight focus groups were held with service providers, health department personnel and policy makers. The study sites were the following: Broadway and Telegraph area is in the old downtown. Lake Merritt is also off the downtown and is a congregation point for homosexual contact or men who have sex with men (MSMs). Fruitvale is the predominantly Latino district of East Oakland and is a congregation point for IDUs and sex workers. The Lower Bottom is in West Oakland.

The initial field assessment focused on the types of persons at risk, where high-risk takers congregate, and the time of day or night that they are present. The underlying assumption of this approach was that the causes of the HIV/AIDS epidemic in Alameda County were evident in publicly accessible behaviors, i.e., the publicly accessible behaviors were indicators of similar behaviors that were occurring even more widely in private settings.

The specific qualitative methods used in the RARE process were:

1. Observations and mapping: Outreach workers trained in ethnography worked in pairs and conducted observations for two hour time intervals, at different times, and recorded their observations. Observing at different times and places, opened opportunities for insight into the organization of public HIV/AIDS risk-taking and the factors that impact it.
2. Intercept interviews: Outreach observers interviewed individuals whom they encountered who either engaged in a particular HIV/AIDS high-risk behavior or were knowledgeable of it. These interviews provided insight into the motivations for high-risk HIV/AIDS behaviors and the social characteristics of the individuals who engage in them. These interviews were tape recorded and transcribed.
3. Key informant interviews: Outreach observers selected individuals who were particularly knowledgeable about MSMs, IDUs, and sex traders' movements, motives, ways of operation as well as the efficiency and effectiveness of prevention services. They were interviewed in-depth, one-on-one and their responses were also tape recorded and transcribed.
4. Focus groups: The team leaders and outreach investigators conducted in-depth focus group interviews with individuals drawn from each group of HIV/AIDS risk takers and outreach workers who have worked closely with HIV/AIDS risk takers in the four observation areas. Stakeholders were also interviewed to learn their insights regarding the HIV/AIDS epidemic in Oakland and the county. These interviews were also tape recorded and transcribed.

The observation, focus groups, intercept and key informant interview transcript notes were all carefully reviewed. Information that was relevant to answering these project's key questions was noted. If the same point was made independently by at least three different participants in any of the data sources (intercept interviews, key informant interviews, focus groups, and observation) it was taken as a finding. There was a second source of insight into the four sets of questions. We had weekly de-briefing and training meetings where each team would present overviews of their findings and notes from the prior week. Team members were questioned by the investigators and other team members about points they might have overlooked in their notes as well as important things said to them that they might not have focused on. These meetings constituted ongoing focus groups of the team as a whole and were taperecorded. The following are our key findings based upon a triangulation of data.

Findings

Men Who Have Sex with Men (MSMs)

Finding 1: Over the past two years, there has been a decline in sites appropriate for anonymous sex in the Lake Merritt and Telegraph and Broadway areas. There is evidence that new sites are emerging in more distant locations.

Scrubs and bushes have been cut and removed around the Lake and a new lighting system has been installed. As a result, hidden locations where MSM sex can take place have been significantly reduced. In the downtown Telegraph Avenue and Broadway area, well-known "bookstores" and "video-shops" continue to provide locations for anonymous sex. But the surrounding area is rapidly changing with renovations and restorations of buildings and new businesses moving in. This new activity is both isolating MSM-sex locations and calling attention to them.

Finding 2: There are MSMs who are HIV-positive and who actively engage in unprotected sex with other men, even after disclosing their HIV-positive status.

MSMs are a diverse population with regard to HIV/AIDS warnings. For some, warnings of the danger of engaging in unprotected sex with HIV-positive individuals are being forgotten and ignored as the threat of HIV/AIDS has become routine. There are some HIV-positive and negative MSMs alike who seem to be resistant to the HIV/AIDS prevention message.

Finding 3: MSMs are developing more long-term relationships with drive-in client-partners.

Observations and key informants report increasing numbers of affluent men driving into the Lake Merritt and Telegraph-Broadway area to have sex with other men. The men working these areas "interviewed" their client-partners and passed the information to our outreach observers. Client-partners mostly live in distant suburbs; many are married and have families, and are professionals. These men pay well and in doing so provide a source of income for indigent MSMs. A number of these encounters have become long-term where there are regular meetings and occasionally the paid MSM is taken away for a weekend, or for several days at a time. It is reported that a number of the indigent MSMs are HIV-positive and that a number of the paying MSMs pay extra not to use condoms.

Finding 4: Observers noted increasing numbers of adolescent MSMs engaged in sexual exchanges for money and/or drugs.

Informants spoke of young men who were available for sex for money. One outreach team interviewed such a young man. He and the others reported that homeless gay and bisexual adolescent men from other states and cities are befriended by older men. These men then bring them to Oakland to work as male prostitutes to have sex with other MSMs.

Finding 5: Heterosexual and MSM sexual networks overlap.

There are women who drive into East Oakland, and the Lake Merritt and Telegraph-Broadway areas and employ MSMs as male prostitutes. There are homeless heterosexual men who have survival sex with MSMs for money; and there is sex reported between MSMs, and MSMs and women at suburb rave parties.

We learned about women who employ MSMs as prostitutes because they are particularly attracted to the adolescent MSMs. We have no idea how extensive this is, but these women's sexual preference in Oakland came up several times in the interviews. We have known about homeless heterosexual survival sex for some time, but not in the context of sex with MSMs. The new findings are about "raves" in south county (Hayward and San Leandro). Oakland and suburban MSMs and heterosexual young people use drugs, in particular ecstasy, and have unprotected sex with each other.

Finding 6: MSMs reported that there were no medical services available to them and that the staff at existing medical facilities was unwelcoming and hostile to them.

This was the most consistent finding regarding MSMs. There is virtually a universal perception that they cannot seek medical services or get tested for HIV or anything else in Oakland medical facilities because of the negative attitudes of medical service providers toward them. Also, medical services are not available when they need them after hours.

Findings for IDUs

Finding 7: The sites for public drug use and dealing have been drastically constrained and are all well-known to the police. As a result, drug use and dealing are now out of sight, beepers and cell phones are used to deal drugs, and drug prices have increased.

A combination of gentrification, resident outrage at crack dealing, and effective police service have driven injection drug users off the streets in Fruitvale, and in East and West Oakland. Bars, clubs, inexpensive restaurants, and remote out-of-sight locations are the new congregation points. Drug dealing is now even more covert. Users arrange arbitrary locations to buy and sell drugs by pagers and cellular phones. In the past decade, the price of drugs has also gone up.

> Finding 8: There are new injector congregation sites in the low-income areas of South County and north of Oakland in Contra Costa County.

The constraint on congregation sites in Oakland due to gentrification and policing, and the general displacement of the poor from the city has implications for street identifiable IDUs. New IDU congregation sites were reported in the lowest-income areas of Hayward and San Leandro. The same potential exists for new emerging locations in the lowest-income pockets of Contra Costa County as well.

> Finding 9: There are new injectors who consist of former crack users and young people who sniff heroin. Some are as young as thirteen and fourteen years old.

The legions of crack cocaine addicts in the early 1990s did not disappear. Many of them sought to temper their cocaine addiction by using heroin. Cocaine stimulates the central nervous system, while heroin depresses it. As a result, crack addicts also have become addicted to heroin. As their tolerance for heroin increased so did their addiction. They are now injecting heroin and cocaine, and many still use crack. In the same way, young people who were initially turned off to crack after observing what it did to older users, snorted heroin. At first, they avoided both the ravages of crack and the needle use of heroin. But as they became addicted to heroin, their tolerance to heroin increased. Soon, they too began injecting heroin.

> Finding 10: The drugs used by IDUs, primarily heroin and cocaine, vary in purity during each month and are often contaminated with infectious materials.

The purity can range from a very low percent to almost 100%. The drugs are reported to be stronger around the first and fifteenth of the month, when social support checks are mailed.

> Finding 11: Injection drug users are now poly-drug users. Besides alcohol, they also use crack cocaine and PCP regularly. They use whatever drugs are available.

Five years ago, heroin and cocaine injectors were distinct populations. These who used both drugs, "speed-balls," were a distinct minority. It is well known that cocaine users have to inject more often than heroin users—5 to 10 times versus 1 to 3. As a result, the cocaine injectors and speed-ballers had higher rates of HIV infection. Now it is reported from a variety of sources that most injectors speed-ball as a matter of routine, and smoke crack cocaine as well. When heroin and cocaine are either not readily available or diluted in purity, injectors will use whatever other drugs are available, notably PCP.

> Finding 12: Some Oakland police use the needle exchange sites to investigate clients and to confiscate used and new exchanged needles.

There are laws against needle possession in some parts of the United States and needles are not made available to addicts by prescription in Oakland. As a result, there are not enough needles in circulation for the number of addicts and the frequency that they inject drugs. If needles are not properly cleaned, injectors end up sharing potential HIV-contaminated needles. The purpose of needle exchanges is to exchange potentially HIV-contaminated needles for clean and unused needles on a one-for-one basis. It has been demonstrated in a series of prior studies that injectors who regularly use the exchange significantly reduce their risk of HIV infection. It has also been reported that police officers have tossed confiscated needles into garbage cans and sewers.

> Finding 13: IDUs reported that there were no medical services available to them and that the staff at existing medical facilities was unwelcoming and hostile to them.

As with MSMs, there is a virtually universal perception that IDUs cannot seek medical services or get tested for HIV or anything else in Oakland because of the attitudes of medical service providers toward them. They report being refused services at Highland Hospital and other facilities, skipped over in waiting room lines until all others have been served, and told that they must first be sober for least a month to receive care. Also clinic-based medical services are not available to them when they are most likely to seek care after hours.

Findings for Sex Traders

> Finding 14: The primary clients of HIV-positive women who trade sex for money and/or drugs drive into East and West Oakland from suburban communities.

Our starting assumption was that the clients of sex traders lived in the areas where sex trading took place. There is no evidence to suggest that anything has changed regarding local clients, but we did get a number of reports that the primary money in sex trading comes from clients who drive into East and West Oakland from suburban communities and pay well. Some will pay extra money for their sex traders not to use condoms.

> Finding 15: There are HIV-positive sex traders who trade sex near Bay Area Rapid Transit (BART) stations and who ride BART to the end of the line and trade sex for money in migrant worker camps.

BART sex clients leave the station and engage sex traders in the parking lots and nearby bushes, return to the station and continue their journey. There are others who ride BART out to the end of the line on weekends and are driven to migrant worker camps. There, they trade sex for money and make a week's income.

> Finding 16: There are women on public support who are neither drug users nor regular sex traders who occasionally engage in survival sex.

There are a number of reports from outreach workers of non-addict women who occasionally take sex clients. They are generally on some combination of welfare to support their children and find that their payments do not cover the escalating costs of rent and living in Oakland. To make ends meet toward the end of the month, they go into the streets and trade sex for money.

Recommendations

The following recommendations are courses of action that are known to be effective in addressing the HIV implications of each finding. There are findings for MSMs, IDUs and sex traders that overlap. In those cases, the recommendation is applicable across HIV risk groups.

Recommendation 1.

Upgrade street outreach from a focus primarily on street contacts and education to more specific case management emphasizing work with specific highest risk-taking clients to get them to reduce their HIV/AIDS risk.

Recommendation 2.

There is a need for more service providers and outreach workers who are better trained in reaching and working with high-risk groups. The training should be standardized and have the capacity to teach service providers to tailor outreach to specific populations and activities in the area. There is a need to cover new public sites, and to reach new and existing MSMs, IDUs, crack users and sex traders at times when they are most accessible.

Recommendation 3.

Increase and continue to support the number of harm-reduction sites that offer needle exchange, and expand the services at all the sites to include secondary prevention with people who are HIV-positive.

Recommendation 4.

Have outreach workers specifically dedicated to finding and bringing into HIV/AIDS-prevention services young MSMs and IDUs.

Recommendation 5.

HIV/AIDS-prevention outreach workers should expand their services to include women who engage in survival sex and do not identify as sex workers.

Recommendation 6.

There is a need for dedicated shelters for young substance abusers (alcohol, heroin, crack, etc.) and adolescent and young-adult MSMs to get them off the streets and out of risk.

Recommendation 7.

Expand and create high-quality drug treatment to include residential medicated detoxification facilities that are available on demand. This will require that space be made available to outreach workers to bring drug abusers including crack cocaine users into treatment at any time.

Recommendation 8.

There is a need for a combination of stationary sites and mobile medical vans to provide services to MSMs, sex workers, IDUs and crack users at off-hours and where HIV high risk-takers congregate at night.

Recommendation 9.

Have at county hospitals and clinics trained and culturally competent admissions officers, community liaisons and counselors where IDUs, crack users and MSMs are likely to seek services.

Recommendation 10.

There is a need to educate the police force about HIV/AIDS and the role that outreach and needle exchanges play in prevention. This would also call for establishing cooperative relations between outreach professionals and the police. It must be explained to needle exchange clients that they cannot come to the exchange with drugs or any illegal contraband other than used needles for exchange.

Recommendation 11.

Have the police stop confiscating needles and condoms from outreach workers and exchange clients at and near the exchange sites. They should also learn to dispose of needles properly, and not to investigate exchange clients at exchange sites.

Recommendation 12.

Have prevention media campaigns on major streets, in BART and at other public transportation systems warning and educating of the HIV/AIDS risk of drug use, and unprotected sex. There is a need to reach at least two audiences. They are street identified HIV high risk-takers and their paying clients.

Recommendation 13.

Have outreach workers serve BART stations and their surrounding areas during off-hours.

Response to Study and Recommendations

In 2001, the study was well received by the Alameda County Public Health Department, the HIV Prevention Planning Council, The Health Services Planning Council and the African American State of Emergency Task Force. Initial critical comments were that much of what was found was already known and that the main recommendations have been proposed before and would be expensive to implement. The Rapid Assessment report and recommendations were reviewed by the Health Department and the planning councils to be integrated into their ongoing efforts. But some members of these various councils and groups did not see the Rapid Assessment and its report as technical assistance to them, but as a competing plan for implementation and funding that could potentially upstage the planning and advocacy they had been engaged in.

While the Rapid Assessment was being conducted, the community-based AIDS service organizations, specifically targeting African Americans, worked with Congresswoman Barbara Lee's office and substantially increased federal funding by some $8 million to their network of organizations. Also prior to the release of the RARE report, all of the planning councils and African American task force of agencies formed the Joint Planning Council of Alameda County. The Joint Council pointed out that, even with increased federal funding, there was still insufficient money to mount an effective HIV-prevention effort. So an increase of $500,000 in county funds was requested from the County Board of Supervisors as a 3% cost of living adjustment to existing direct services. The request was granted. The Joint Council also requested $300,000 from Tobacco Tax Settlement money to expand the local needle exchanges. This is an important and effective harm-reduction effort that federal funds are prohibited from funding. This request was granted as well.

Based on the Oakland RARE findings, $126,676 of county direct services money from the State of California was designed for a pilot night outreach program targeting HIV high-risk populations in Central, West, and East Oakland, and areas in Fremont, south of Oakland. In addition, based upon supplemental funds from the U.S. Office of AIDS as a follow-up to RARE, the county was provided money to recruit HIV high risk-takers late at night and conduct HIV tests. This was to test a central RARE finding that the highest HIV risk-takers and those who are HIV infected are more accessible and congregate at night after county clinics are closed and after most outreach workers have gone home. The Joint Council also made a recommendation directly related to RARE. They asked that the county health department staff do a cost analysis of the recommendations identified in the RARE report. The Council saw the recommendations as reflecting three priority funding areas—improving and expanding prevention outreach, increasing access to drug treatment, and expanding prevention case management for HIV-positive persons. Two years after RARE (2003), this cost analysis is still not complete.

Everyone involved in HIV prevention in Alameda counties agree that there is not enough money to mount an effective prevention effort. When one compares Alameda County's HIV service budgets with those of San Francisco and San Diego, the deficiency is apparent. Both of these other California counties have more AIDS cases than Alameda County, but they also have proportionally more money for services as indicated in the following table.

Table 8.3: HIV/AIDS Service Budget in 2000 by California Counties with the Most AIDS Cases

County	AIDS Cases Thru 12/00	Alameda Cases as ratio of:	HIV/AIDS Services Budget	Alameda $ as ratio of:	Difference in $ ratio to Case ratio
San Francisco	27,332	.219	$64,000,000	.156	.71
San Diego	15,000	.400	$37,680,000	.265	.66
Alameda	6,000		$10,000,000		

In 2000, Alameda County had 22% of the number of AIDS cases of San Francisco and 40% of the cases of San Diego. But Alameda County had only 16% of San Francisco's and 27% of San Diego's AIDS service budgets. This works out to be 71 cents of every dollar San Francisco spent per AIDS case and 66 cents of every dollar San Diego spent per AIDS case. The disparity is worse on a per capita population basis. Spending under Ryan White Title I money for

San Francisco in fiscal year 1999 totaled $4,098 per AIDS case compared to $2,218 in the Oakland EMA (Alameda and Contra Costa Counties). Clearly, spending either per AIDS case or per capita population in Alameda County is lower than in San Francisco or San Diego (Council 2001).

With regard to funding, Alameda County health officials point out that they cannot spend any more money on HIV prevention. There are other crises to address that are even more under-funded than the AIDS crisis and affect a larger number of residents, such as declining pre-natal care, and rising cancer, stroke and heart disease rates—also heavily concentrated among African Americans. Off the record, federal and state officials say they are reluctant to put more money directly into Alameda County because the county has not maximized funding through existing federal programs. In other words, there are more dollars the county can get potentially if it can manage to apply for them.

In comparison, neither San Francisco nor San Diego has a larger African American population than Alameda County. Nor do they have an AIDS epidemic driven largely by increasing levels of HIV infections among African Americans. The epidemic in Alameda County is well along and in hard-to-reach sub-populations. But there is a more basic issue as to whether Alameda County could get a handle on its AIDS epidemic, even if it spent the equivalent amounts of money as San Francisco and San Diego. Given the extent to which AIDS is increasing in Alameda County, it might take even more money per AIDS case or per capita to reverse HIV infection rates than in San Francisco or San Diego.

A greater barrier to effective prevention in Alameda County is organizational rather than financial. It turns out that a RARE study of county services and organizations may be as critical a need as a RARE study of HIV high-risk populations. Despite a committed public health department and a rich network of community-based organizations, HIV prevention and care are not well coordinated in Alameda County. For example, there is overlap in responsibility that has led to conflicting roles between outreach workers in community-based agencies and county-based case managers. With regard to the highest HIV risk groups in Alameda County, clinic services are offered at the wrong times (8 a.m. to 5 p.m.) and to the wrong people (comparatively HIV low-risk groups who utilize facilities). Services are offered by people who are not particularly interested in serving HIV high risk takers (injectors, homosexuals, sex traders, crack addicts and the homeless). These potential clients are more often black, poor, come with "attitudes" and negative expectations, and are interpersonally difficult to deal with. The only people in the entire system of prevention and services who have a track record of reaching and effectively dealing with the highest HIV risk-takers are community-based outreach workers.

Probably the single greatest organizational barrier to effective services and prevention in Alameda County is that public health is separate from hospital and clinic services. The Public Health Department is separate from Behavioral Health Services which runs hospitals, clinics and drug treatment. In addition, most outreach and prevention educational services are contracted out to community-based agencies by the Public Health Department. So there are three separate organizations responsible for addressing the AIDS epidemic in Alameda County—the Public Health Department, Behavioral Health and community-based organizations. An effective prevention campaign to reverse the AIDS epidemic would require flawless cooperation and seamless coordination among all three sectors. While these sectors spend a great deal of time and energy in meetings to coordinate their services, there are significant gaps that are obvious to outsiders.

The gaps in organization seriously compromise the community's response to AIDS. First, community-based and Public Health Department outreach workers are dependent upon referring HIV high risk-takers to health clinics and treatment programs run by Alameda County Behavioral Health. If their clients are not well received and do not work well with the clinics and treatment staff, clients come back to the streets with experiences and stories that discourage others from seeking care. Then outreach services are compromised; they have no place to refer clients. All of the high-risk groups interviewed in the RARE study reported that they felt unwelcome, disrespected, and poorly treated at the county clinics and hospitals. HIV high-risk persons avoided these facilities and the services they offered as much as possible—until they were seriously ill and had no choice. While the Public Health Department is directly responsible for addressing the AIDS epidemic in the county, it has no direct authority to address the clinic staff treatment of high-risk clients, hours of operation or where services are rendered. Behavioral Health Care is in charge of these matters.

Second, within Behavioral Health Care there is opposition to harm-reduction measures essential to reducing HIV risk among actively using drug abusers. The county's treatment programs will have nothing to do with actively using drug abusers, just like health clinic staff wish to avoid them. Opposition to active drug users includes any risk-reduction outreach services such as needle exchange. Short of a commitment to being clean and sober, active drug users are unwanted in Behavioral Health Care.

Third, most outreach and educational services moneys that come to the Public Health Department are sub-contracted to outside venders, most of whom are community-based agencies. This is because the Public Health Department is highly regulated. For example, all contracts or amendments to contracts must be approved by the County Board of Supervisors, even if the funding is external and not from county sources. It can take months to get a contract approved regardless of how time sensitive it might be. And the hours that staff work, and what they can and cannot do, is highly regulated by civil service rules. So for flexibility and rapid response, lower administrative costs, and to get technical capacity not on staff, services are sub-contracted.

But structural conflict is built into the relationship between sub-contractors and the Public Health Department, because the same burdensome reporting and oversight requirements that necessitated outsourcing in the first place are extended to sub-contractors. This is particularly problematic when department staff has no sense of what is required to work effectively in communities with hard to reach and potentially dangerous sub-populations. It takes time and creativity to reach covert HIV high risk takers such as injectors, young economically marginalized black men, and men who have sex with men. It requires developing trust and a process to identify and train the people who can work best with them. Therefore, phases in effective outreach projects may take more or less time than is specified in a contract and may require exact steps not initially specified. Subcontractors report that department reporting requirements can sometimes be more burdensome and problematic than actually doing the work.

Fourth, community-based outreach organizations have specific constituencies that they direct their services to and are most skilled at working with. So there are agencies that work primarily with gay and bisexual men, or adolescents, or women and in particular communities. So people who do not fit the agency's target group do not get reached or served. If an injector is gay and bisexual or is a Latino adolescent sex trader or a woman who is not a drug abuser but who engages in survival sex, he or she falls through the cracks in service. No one outreach organization addresses these specific identities or works in all the neighborhoods where there are risk-takers. This means that most community-based agencies are not organized or diverse enough to reach the complex and diversity groups of HIV risk-takers in Alameda County. So they are marginally effective in the field. Furthermore, because of the ambivalence of Behavioral Health Services toward their HIV high risk clients, community-based agencies are attempting to duplicate existing health services in their programs and in the field. These are mobile van-based health services and mini-health clinics at needle exchange sites. Outreach workers also have to get their clients housing, food, legal services, employment and children's services in order to motivate them to reduce their HIV risks. Outreach workers are not trained or funded to do any of these things.

In effect, the Public Health Department cannot be held responsible for essential services and resources that should be forthcoming from Behavioral Health Care. What it could do is maximize federal and state funding. Community-based agencies cannot replace services that should come from Behavioral Health nor can they work effectively while being restrained by administrative rigidity from the Health Department. It is not just HIV high risk takers in Alameda County who have to change their behaviors to reduce their HIV risks and the AIDS epidemic in the county. It also will require behavioral change on the part of the county and community agencies to address their organizational barriers to effective outreach and health services.

References

Council, A. C. J. P. (2001) *Report of the Joint Planning Council to the Alameda County Board of Supervisors. Oakland.*

Daniels, D. H. (1980). *Pioneer Urbanites: A social and cultural history of Black San Francisco.* Philadelphia: Temple University Press.

Hayes, E. (1972). *Power Structure and Urban Policy: Who rules in Oakland?* New York: McGraw-Hill.

Hunter, F. (1964). *Housing discrimination in Oakland, California: A study prepared for the Oakland Mayor's Committee on Full Opportunity and the Council of Social Planning, Alameda County.* Berkeley: Floyd Hunter Company.

U.S. Census Bureau (1980) *County and City Data Book.* Washington: U.S. Government Printing Office.

Chapter 9

The AIDS Epidemic in Palm Beach County, Florida

Karen Dodge
Barbara Feeney

Selection of Palm Beach County

Twenty cities were originally eligible for this assistance under RARE. Eleven cities requested the assistance. Palm Beach County, while not a city, was one of the eleven first-tier sites selected for implementation. The reason for selection is that as of December 2000, a total of 7,643 residents of Palm Beach County had been diagnosed with AIDS. Sixty-three percent (4,815) of these AIDS cases were black and 7% (535) were Hispanic.

The Advisory Board, using zip code-based HIV incidence data from the previous twelve months, identified four general areas in the county that appeared to meet the selection criteria of being areas in which HIV was having a disproportionate impact on the minority community. These four areas were initially identified as North Coastal, South Coastal, Central Coastal, and Western. Of the 3,388 presumed alive adult AIDS cases in the county as of December 31, 2000, 65% (2,202) were black and 8% (271) were Hispanic.

Through subsequent focus groups and individual interviews documented in the detailed findings, specific "hot spots" in the four areas were identified more precisely as specific road intersections. While these intersections are precisely defined and documented in the findings, the terms North Coastal, South Coastal, Central Coastal, and Western were retained in the narrative to avoid creating the misleading impression that the specific intersections are the only locations where HIV transmission is occurring.

The Target Areas

Although many factors were considered when selecting these areas, the major determining factor was a mid-July 1997 epidemiological report of HIV infection in Palm Beach County by zip code. The zip codes with the highest number of HIV cases reported were considered the highest priority areas. According to the Florida Department of Health HIV/AIDS Reporting System (HARS), there were four zip code areas with high rates of HIV infection. They were 33404 referred to as North Coastal, 33460 which is Central Coastal, 33444 which is South Coastal, and 33430 Western. These four areas are characterized by high levels of poverty, substance abuse and high-risk sexual behavior relating to HIV/AIDS.

Another factor considered was anecdotal information alluding to hidden pockets of migrant populations (e.g., Haitians and Guatemalans) who lacked knowledge of HIV risk or infection or who, for a variety of reasons, might not be receiving treatment. The Advisory Board listened to anecdotal reports of people in these areas who had never been tested and had "fallen through the cracks" of the current surveillance system or had been tested, but were not receiving appropriate treatment.

While residents of the western portions of the county had already been the subjects of state and federal research regarding HIV/AIDS, many other subpopulations in the county had not been studied by research scientists at all. Therefore, to begin to lessen the gaps in knowledge about some of these other populations, this study included specific coastal populations in need of more effective prevention and treatment interventions.

A total of 1,439 cases of HIV were diagnosed in Palm Beach County between July 31, 1997, and September 2000. Ten zip codes accounted for 1,054 (71.3%) of all the cases in the county. Of those ten zip codes, four were selected as areas to begin implementing the RARE methodology. Two zip codes, 33401 and 33407, which also have a high number and percentage of cases, were not selected as RARE sites because they are currently being studied through other initiatives. The four zip codes designated as the four RARE areas accounted for 571 (38.3%) of all the cases in Palm Beach County during the baseline period. For the purpose of this study, these four areas were named North Coastal, Central Coastal, South Coastal, and Western, respectively. This wide geographic distribution was intended to identify a broad range of previously unidentified or underserved high-risk populations.

Palm Beach County RARE Project Goals

The overall goals of Palm Beach County's RARE project include:

- Reducing HIV/AIDS morbidity and mortality;
- Affirming the many existing efforts and current intervention strategies being utilized in Palm Beach County;
- Increasing and enhancing current responses to HIV spectrum disease;
- Contributing to HIV/AIDS prevention and medical treatment through a directed investigation of high-risk populations using research con-

ducted by high-risk populations (i.e., injection drug users; men who have sex with men; minority males who have sex with males; minority females who have sex with men who have sex with men; individuals who exchange sex for drugs and/or money, etc.);

- Working in partnership with the local communities to gather information about treatment and prevention availability and effectiveness;
- Presenting detailed information from people affected by a specific health problem who are seldom included in traditional research designs and implementation, yet are the people most affected by these problems.

Palm Beach Methodology

A unique feature of RARE is its overall approach to data collection and analysis. Rapid assessments utilize a detective-like approach, which tends to neutralize any cultural or political incentives to deny the existence of certain activities, such as substance abuse and prostitution. The advantage of rapid assessment methods over other social science approaches is that they encourage the constant crosschecking of information from various sources. This helps uncover information that may be invisible to traditional methods of observation.

For example, the reports of community experts can be checked against the descriptions in direct observations. Investigators work inductively and build their conclusions or theories from the ground up by collating and checking from a wide array of sources. This is called "grounded theory", based on "idiographic" or "inductive" theoretical construction. This model aims at explanation through the enumeration of all the motivations and contributing factors in a given action or situation. The purpose of this type of research is to understand a particular situation as fully as possible.

This research model also recognizes that, to be accurate and meaningful, researchers must view and describe a problem within its social, cultural, religious, political, and historical contexts. Thus, rapid assessments move across several levels of investigation in order to identify different potential levels of intervention

The five strategies described in this section were used to collect data to answer the research questions in this study. They were focus groups, key informant/community expert interviews, geo-mapping, direct observation, and rapid assessment surveys/street intercepts.

Findings

The primary HIV risk groups in the North Coastal area were substance abusers/ addicts, prostitutes and homosexuals most of whom were African American. In the Central Coastal area those at risk were primarily Guatemalan migrant workers and other Hispanics. We found primarily Haitians, prostitutes, drug addicts and African Americans at risk in the South Coast. African American substance abusers/addicts and prostitutes and immigrants from the Caribbean, and Central and South America, were the primary HIV risk-takers in the Western area.

The Fundamental Elements of Time and Place

In all four sites, time and place were influential factors in HIV risk, prevention, treatment, and access to services. For example, some Haitians and Guatemalans, especially those from agrarian cultures who have low levels of literacy, or have recently immigrated to the U.S., may be unfamiliar with the concept of "telling time" by a watch or a clock. Members of both populations may, instead, "tell time" in reference to an *event* rather than numbers on a clock. This is a critical factor to consider when scheduling appointments, expecting drug adherence, prescribing medications, or arranging for the delivery of social and/or medical services.

Additionally, in the Southern Coastal and Central Coastal areas, study participants reported being afraid to go to the Department of Health's main HIV clinic because the then-named U.S. Immigration and Naturalization Service (INS) is located the same building. Many Haitians and Guatemalans reported fear of arrest and deportation. Thus, the proximity of patient care services to the INS appeared significantly to impede access to care.

Beliefs, Attitudes and Practices Relating to HIV/AIDS

At each site, study participants reported a variety of beliefs, attitudes, and practices relating to HIV/AIDS. Factors such as religious beliefs, medical practices, alternative therapies, gender-related issues, and stigmatization generated different approaches within each culture.

For example, reports of social and familial rejection were common among study participants. Testing, diagnosis, and treatment of HIV continue to be highly stigmatized within the targeted communities. HIV-infected members of some target populations stated that, in their communities they are considered to be sinners or that their HIV infection is a punishment from God.

A significant disparity in power between men and women was observed within all four data collection sites, but most prominently among recent Haitian and Guatemalan immigrants. Unprotected heterosexual sex, prostitution, and drug use were common themes relating to a disparity of power between men and women. Providers of clinical services reported a relatively high level of these risk behaviors and factors among Haitians and Guatemalans.

Variations in Language and Literacy

Study participants at three sites indicated that the inability to speak, read, and write English presented an obstacle to HIV prevention and treatment services. For example, while some Guatemalans speak Spanish, most speak one of twenty-six Mayan Indian dialects. Unfortunately, many health care workers try to speak to them in Spanish while attempting to explain a complex HIV treatment protocol, or the concept of transmission of bodily fluids.

The Mixing of Alcohol, Drugs and Sex

In all four areas, study participants reported an interaction between alcohol, drugs, sex and HIV risk. The various populations interact, and HIV risk is highest wherever high-risk sex and substance abuse meet. As in all the major themes, there is variation in the relationship between substance abuse and sex. For example, it appears that within the Guatemalan and Haitian communities, alcohol and drugs are used to facilitate high-risk sex behavior. In contrast, within the African American communities on the coast and in the western part of the county, it appears that sex is performed to obtain drugs. Underlying virtually all risk behaviors in all the target populations are issues related to poverty and economic incentives that promote the sex-for-drugs and drugs-for-sex economy.

Prevention and Patient Care Services

There was a general lack of awareness or absence of services in the intervention zones. There were two major dimensions to the issue of services. First, study participants indicated inadequate access to preventive and patient care services in the target areas. Second, providers described a dichotomy between prevention and patient care services. Some prevention providers were critical of patient care services, citing instances of perceived poor service delivery and an unwelcoming attitude toward patients from the hot spots. Likewise, some patient care providers reported being unaware of the efforts and successful outcomes of prevention services among target populations.

Recommendations

On July 20, 2001, the RARE Community Advisory Board recommended that the Palm Beach County Department of Health convene a committee to consider the findings of this report in realigning existing resources, and refining and prioritizing the following recommendations and strategies:

Recommendation 1: Demonstrate the continued commitment of Palm Beach County to HIV prevention and clinical care activities by taking a leadership role in identifying and securing additional funding to address and implement the recommendations.

Strategies:

1. Commit and/or provide through the county, the mechanism to secure additional funding to support harm reduction and HIV care and prevention outreach initiatives, including, but not limited to:

- The dissemination of wound care items,
- Water and condom distribution,
- Syringe/needle kits,
- Expanded HIV/AIDS, STD and family planning, counseling, testing, and referral services,
- Expanded HIV primary care, case management, and other supportive services.

2. Dedicate and secure funding through the Board of County Commissioners and through each municipality to provide HIV liaisons with local, state, and national HIV/AIDS networks.

3. Provide funding and other support to ensure organizations targeting high-risk populations have the technical assistance necessary for capacity building, preparing them for future expansion.

Recommendation 2: Educate county and city commissioners, community leadership, and all health care providers in the county about high-risk communities and the special needs of their residents regarding HIV/AIDS prevention and treatment. Emphasize the importance of commitment to a systemic and systematic planning process for change.

Strategies:

1. Establish an HIV/AIDS Round Table Forum comprised of elected officials and administrators from the four RARE team sites, the RARE ethnographers and team leaders, Department of Health officials, HIV-related service providers, other health care providers, and other stakeholders necessary to the development and implementation of effective solutions. The inclusion of representatives of economic development and educational services is imperative to developing comprehensive and meaningful change.

2. Integrate ongoing HIV/AIDS care and prevention as an integral part of Palm Beach County's community agencies that provide services to the targeted populations at risk for contracting HIV. Such entities include, but are

not limited to:

- City of West Palm Beach Community Development Office
- Grantees for Housing Opportunities for People with AIDS (HOPWA)
- Palm Beach County School District
- Palm Beach County Sheriff's Office
- Palm Beach County Mental Health Board

3. Issue a county "Call for Action on HIV/AIDS Prevention and Medical Care" that demands partnerships between community service providers and city, county, state and federal agencies, and that requests both programmatic and fiscal resources.

Recommendation 3: Urge elected officials, local planners, providers, colleges, universities, and other policy makers to utilize the findings of this report when developing and implementing programs to decrease HIV/AIDS incidence, prevalence, morbidity, and mortality among high-risk populations.

Strategies:

1. Establish an advisory group to develop and/or review national and local programs that provide peer-based HIV training and mentoring.

2. Form a research collaborative with colleges and universities to explore and examine HIV/AIDS literature, interventions, policies, program evaluations, and analyses.

3. Provide local training updates on a quarterly basis for all involved in HIV/AIDS service provision at a local college and/or university. Offer class credits or credentials for successful participation.

4. Disseminate the findings of this ethnographic report to local and regional educational institutions to develop support and feedback.

Recommendation 4: Increase the availability of and access to HIV prevention and medical care for African American, Latino, Guatemalan, Haitian, and Caribbean Basin bisexuals and homosexuals within the identified risk pockets.

Strategies:

1. Develop and sustain street-level interventions which are based on epidemiologic and ethnographic trends. Evaluate these interventions on an ongoing basis. These interventions should concentrate on hidden populations living in or frequenting the RARE-identified risk pockets.

2. Contact, establish, and/or make services accessible through African American and Latino gay organizations that are targeted to behaviors occurring in the risk pockets as well as the risk behavior initiation points that are identified in this report. These services need to be formally linked with opportunities for HIV testing and counseling.

3. Mobilize HIV prevention and medical outreach services. Services must be provided in non-traditional settings and at non-traditional hours (not just 9–5) or days (not just Monday-Friday) to effectively reach targeted populations in their geographic pockets.

Recommendation 5: Establish targeted funding to address the HIV/AIDS barriers related to minority communities as identified in the Palm Beach County RARE report. This targeted funding should be used to fund minority organizations in order to meet HIV prevention and patient care needs.

Strategies:

1. Encourage collaboration between established HIV/AIDS providers, public health, community-based organizations, and emerging minority agencies.

2. Provide adequate funding for HIV education for providers, especially in areas that are identified as having high concentrations of high-risk behaviors and vulnerable individuals.

3. Reinstate HIV/AIDS prevention and patient care services in the labor camps.

4. Form a collaborative of minority organizations that can develop proposals to apply for grants and contracts on a unified basis. The collaborative should establish rapport with well-established agencies that will provide accurate data upon request.

Recommendation 6: Identify a funding source to conduct additional investigational studies of specific geographic areas having high concentrations of individuals engaging in high-risk behaviors.

Strategies:

1. Obtain funding or make opportunities available to implement the RARE methodology in other risk pockets in Palm Beach County.

2. Provide additional funds to increase capacity building efforts to expand the Palm Beach County Minority Network, and provide training and techni-

cal assistance for community-based organizations to facilitate their access to local funding.

3. Identify and encourage collaboration between private sector and public health to maximize the effectiveness of currently available HIV/AIDS funding streams.

Recommendation 7: Provide adequate funding to conduct a countywide public awareness campaign that reaches all of the targeted populations identified in this study. This campaign should be conducted in English, Spanish, several Mayan Indian dialects, Creole, and French, and should address HIV/AIDS prevention and medical care issues, especially for women, infants, and children.

Strategies:

1. Encourage a partnership between the State of Florida, local cultural organizations, the Port of Palm Beach, private enterprises and the public health system to provide the media with information about HIV/AIDS.

2. Recruit Latino, Guatemalan and Haitian volunteers to deliver written, audio, and visual messages relating to HIV/AIDS via the church, radio, and television.

3. Increase funding or utilize available sources to provide educational outreach to the county's public school system, prison systems, substance abuse treatment facilities, mental health agencies, foster care and other child welfare systems, and local government officials.

4. Educate the populations identified in this study that HIV/AIDS is a public health threat and that the upward trend of other sexually transmitted diseases and teen pregnancies are indicators of high rates of HIV risk behavior.

5. Provide educational opportunities for clinical providers regarding people in their caseloads who are at risk

Recommendation 8: Increase the availability and access to HIV prevention and care services for substance abusers, including injection drug users, within the identified target areas.

Strategies:

1. Produce and implement substance abuse interventions that can be introduced and sustained at the street level, based on the ethnographic and epidemiologic trends noted in the study. These interventions need to focus on the hidden and target populations living in or frequenting these risk pockets without diluting current countywide efforts.

2. Make services available through organizations having a proven track record with the populations identified in this project. Services must be targeted to the behaviors occurring in the neighborhoods represented in this report. These services need to be formally linked with opportunities for HIV counseling and testing and primary medical care.

3. Explore implementing a pilot program of harm reduction strategies that includes a needle exchange program designed to combat the spread of HIV through intravenous drug abuse.

4. Establish minority-based substance abuse treatment programs with an outreach component to address HIV and substance abuse among minority clients in urban and rural settings. Additionally, interventions need to be specifically developed to meet the needs of Guatemalan, Haitian, and Latino substance abusers.

Recommendation 9: Require that employees and volunteers of the local health department and all community-based organizations serving clients in communities of color receive diversity and sensitivity training, and training regarding issues related to sexual orientation. Training should be incorporated into employee orientation and also provided as in-service training on a regular basis.

Strategies:

1. Encourage a partnership between Palm Beach County and Florida's black colleges and universities to educate incoming students via peer mentoring. Likewise, cultivating a relationship with colleges and universities in Puerto Rico and other Caribbean islands might yield similarly beneficial results.

2. Require all state HIV/AIDS contracts to have a staff training component that includes HIV testing standards, train-the-trainer courses, and AIDS 101. If the agency is a test site, it must conform to all requirements set by the Centers for Disease Control and the State of Florida.

3. Recruit Guatemalan, Spanish-speakers, and Haitian workers to provide HIV/AIDS prevention and intervention services to their respective communities in a culturally appropriate manner.

Recommendation 10: Recruit and train indigenous HIV/AIDS educators to raise awareness of and educate individuals about their own HIV risk, in their own languages and communities.

Strategies:

1. Expand the implementation of HIV education in Palm Beach County

schools, grades K–12.

2. Establish a formal linkage to the Palm Beach County HIV/AIDS Community Planning Partnership.

3. Produce culturally appropriate prevention messages and services, including messages transmitted by radio and posters utilizing visual art and illustration for those who are unable to read.

4. Expand current messages to include individuals who may be at risk but who do not identify themselves at risk (e.g., teens, women, drug addicts).

5. Deliver messages by sources respected and understood by individuals engaging in the identified risk behaviors.

Chapter 10

The Risks of Paradise: Project RARE and the Fight against AIDS in the U.S. Virgin Islands

Agatha Nelson
Patricia R. Todman
Merrill Singer

Introduction

The U.S. Virgin Islands are referred to quixotically in travel guides as "America's tourist paradise"—a place of sun-drenched sandy beaches, magnificent countryside, Danish architecture, and the exotic cultural flavor of the West Indians. They are historically, politically, and culturally distinct from the nearby British Virgin Islands, a separation that dates to the 17th century. But in reality, the U.S. Virgin Islands have become one of the public health battlefields in the global fight against AIDS. Like several other Caribbean islands (Castro and Farmer 2004), the U.S. Virgin Islands (VI) have developed a significant AIDS epidemic. The Centers for Disease Control and Prevention (CDC) ranks the VI fourth in the nation in AIDS incidents. Among women, notably, the VI's AIDS case rate of approximately 30 per 100,000 population is nearly three times the national rate (with 27% of AIDS cases and 47% of combined HIV/AIDS cases among women). By the later part of the year 2000, there were over 400 AIDS cases in the VI, 54% of which had already died (Virgin Islands HIV Community Planning Group 2000).

In response, the people of the VI have mounted an effort to increase AIDS awareness, lower the frequency of risk behavior, and meet the needs of those who are already infected. As part of this effort, the VI HIV Community Planning Group, with the backing of the VI Department of Health and support from the Office of HIV/AIDS Policy of the U.S. Department of Health and Human Services, implemented the VI RARE Project in 2000/2001. This chapter documents this project in the Virgin Islands, its findings on AIDS risk, and the recommendations based on these findings that were developed by those who worked on the project.

The U.S. Virgin Islands: Beyond the Tourist Cruise Ships

Officially, the U.S. VI are comprised of seventy islands of varying sizes totaling 352 square kilometers of land, only four of which are inhabited, the most important of these being St. Thomas, St. Croix, and St. John (a fourth island, Water Island, is inhabited by only about eighty-five families). Because of their place in the U.S. tourist trade, they have higher name recognition than most similar sized islands of the Caribbean.

Collectively the islands of the VI, which lie to the east of Puerto Rico in the Lesser Antilles, have a land mass just about double the size of Washington, D.C. with a population approaching 125,000 people. The ethnic composition is 80% black, 15% white and 5% Hispanic. By place of birth, 81% of the population was born in the West Indies (49% in VI and 32% elsewhere in the Caribbean), 13% were born on the U.S. mainland, and 4% were born in Puerto Rico with the remainder of the population coming from elsewhere in the world, especially Latin America.

The Virgin Islands have been U.S.-owned territory since the islands were purchased from Denmark in 1917, for $25 million in gold with the intent of using them as naval outposts to protect the Panama Canal. In 1932, the Organic Action conferred U.S. citizenship and a limited degree of self-rule for the population of the VI. In 1972, the VI sent their first elected delegation of one non-voting representative to the U.S. Congress. With the emergence of the AIDS epidemic, this representative, along with other member of the Congressional Black Caucus, provided strong support for the Project RARE and for the implementation of the project in the Virgin Islands.

Significantly, while the inhabited islands of the VI have a common social history, they have evolved overlapping, but somewhat (often subtly) differing local cultures and cultural identities. The population of each island has distinct ethnic/racial and socio-demographic characteristics. Thus, Hispanics comprise 20% of the population of St. Croix compared to only 6% of the other two islands; whites make up about 23% of the population of St. John compared to fewer than 9% of the St. Thomas population. While the unemployment rate for the VI generally is comparatively high, unemployment is notably higher on St. Croix than the VI as a whole (12.4% vs. 18.4% respectively at the time of the RARE study). The average proportion of the population living below the federal poverty line is significant (almost 21% at the time of the RARE project), but it is not equally distributed across the three islands, with St. Croix having the highest rate (about 26% at the time of the RARE project). These contrasts have helped to shape the differing profiles of the HIV/AIDS epidemic across the three islands.

Charlotte Amalie, on St. Thomas, the capital of the VI, is one of the most beautiful cities and the heaviest visited cruise ship destinations in the West Indies. But the island of St. Thomas has been dubbed the most "unvirgin" of the Virgin Islands, because of its heavy commercial activity, throngs of cruise ship passengers as well as problems with crack cocaine, other drugs and crime. Over 60% of AIDS cases in the VI have been reported from St. Thomas, although the island only accounts for 49% of the total population of the VI. St. Johns, which lies four miles away just across the Pillsbury Sound from St. Thomas, by contrast, has only 4% of the population and only 1% of the VI AIDS case load. Forty miles to the south and on the other side of a deep ocean trench is St. Croix, the largest of the three islands, which has 47% of the population of the VI and 37% of the AIDS case load.

Implementing Project RARE in the Virgin Islands

The Virgin Island RARE project began in the fall of 2000 with the first presentation by the federal Crisis Team to a joint meeting of the Virgin Island Community Planning Groups (CPGs) which voted during the meeting to endorse the project. The training of the project field team took place during February 2001, with data collection carried out between February and July 2001. The Final Report for the project was presented in September 2001. Unlike most other RARE project sites (Needle et al. 2003), the VI project was not conducted in a single city, but on three separate and differing islands. As noted below, this complex social and geographic environment presented real challenges for the RARE initiative which the local RARE team was able to overcome with extra time for project completion.

Organization of Local Project

The VI RARE project was coordinated through the VI Health Department in conjunction with the VI Community Planning Groups (one for each of the three participating islands). The Health Department Coordinator for the VI RARE project was Patricia Odoms, an independent consultant. Drs. Nelson and Todman were the Co-Field Team coordinators of the project. Field teams were constituted on St. Thomas (3 staff), St. Croix (3 staff), and St. John (4 staff). Field team members were recruited from the staffs of community-based organizations on each of the three islands.

The target groups selected by the Community Planning Groups were substance abusers, heterosexual females with high-risk behaviors, and men having sex with men (MSM). Youth 13–19 years of age, which were identified as a potential target group, were not specifically targeted in the data collection as participants, but the needs and risk behaviors of youth were discussed by other participants. Data collection was directed both to identified individuals in the three vulnerable target groups and to places they congregate as well as to community leaders and service providers. Because of the closet nature of homosexuality in VI, the difficulty of identifying MSM, and the loss of several interviews conducted with MSM on St. Croix, the project has been unable to report any data collected from this target population.

Methods

Data collection methods used in the VI RARE project included key informant interviews, street intercept interviews, focus groups, and observations of high-risk sites and site social mapping. Across the three islands, 82 key informant and street intercept interviews were conducted (36 on St. Thomas, 31 on St. Croix, and 15 on St. John). Of these interviews, 20 were with community leaders, 21 were with service providers, 17 were with members of the targeted vulnerable populations and six were with local cultural experts. Most interviews were audio-recorded, although some participants declined to be taped. The primary interview questions used in the street intercept and focus group interviews were: 1) who in your community is most vulnerable to HIV/AIDS?; 2) where in the community are the places for the highest risk for HIV infection?; 3) what conditions in the community contribute to the spread of AIDS?; 4) what is your familiarity with existing intervention services in the community?; and 5) where should interventions be located in the community? Additionally, four focus groups were held (two on St. Thomas, two on St. Croix). Project staff visited many street (e.g., bars, parks, street corners) high-risk sites and developed social maps of the distribution of risk behaviors. On St. Thomas, observations were conducted at market square, a bar in Smith Bay, and a strip club near St. Peter and Paul Catholic Church. On St. Croix, observations were carried out in several downtown bars in the city of Frederiksted and in the cemetery of the city of Christiansted. Street intercept interviews were conducted during the annual Carnival on St. Thomas. Two questions were asked: 1) during Carnival, when people are out having a good time, what do you see as the greatest risk factors for HIV (what groups are most at risk and why), and 2) what do you think the Health Department STD/HIV/TB program can do better to serve the VI community? These questions were supplemented with related questions and probes in key informant interviews.

Issues and Challenges

From the beginning it was recognized that the Virgin Islands presented some unique challenges for the implementation of the RARE initiative. There is a history of logistic and communication problems with implementing cross-island projects that were also encountered in the Project RARE. While the three participating islands are linked by air or sea transport, travel is costly and time consuming and is affected by weather conditions and other contingencies. Research in the VI is further encumbered by limited resources, including both research equipment and trained research personnel. As a result, the project was completed in seven months rather than the projected four-month period.

The specific challenges faced in implementing the RARE initiative were logistical. Because of the multi-island configuration of the project and the cost of traveling between islands, holding frequent face-to-face, full-staff meetings was not possible. It was therefore difficult to coordinate activities and address problems in gathering data. The Field Team Coordinators split the oversight of the islands with one focusing on St. Croix and the other on St. Thomas and St. John. One consequence of the need for frequent travel was that some data (e.g., interviews with MSMs) were lost in transit. Coordinating schedules for field team members across locations and primary employers also posed difficulties. Additionally, given the small size of the total population of the U.S. VI, identifying part-time field team members with related prior experience was difficult. It was especially difficult finding male field team members.

The VI field team was further hampered by difficulty finding an experienced transcriber and transcription machine, although both were eventually found. Additionally, outreach workers who were recruited to the field team sometimes had difficulty separating their primary role as community-based AIDS prevention workers and their role in RARE as community researchers. Finally, the team faced the challenge that homosexuality is a firmly closeted issue in VI and known homosexuals are subject to significant discrimination. The conservative religiosity of much of the community and a strong emphasis on machismo among men means that homosexuals not only are subject to attacks on the streets, they are routinely preached against from the pulpit with their behavior commonly described as a sin and an abomination. As a result, few people publicly identify themselves as MSMs, and gay organizations and known MSM gathering sites (e.g., gay clubs or bars) do not exist. Being gay is a deeply guarded secret and almost no one would discuss the topic openly. Consequently, the closeted gay community was very reluctant to participate in the RARE assessment process. As noted, this problem was further complicated by the fact that the interviews that were conducted on St. Croix with MSMs were lost in transit to St. Thomas and could not be included in the project database.

All sites across the U.S. have confronted challenges in implementing Project RARE because of its rapid nature and its use of part-time staff with limited prior research experience. The inherent value of the qualitative RARE assessment approach helped to sustain the VI RARE project over its seven months of operation because it identifies gaps in the existing AIDS prevention system and translates these shortcomings into achievable recommendations.

Key Findings

Field Observation and Social Mapping

The field teams on the three islands conducted observations of areas that were designated by participants as high-risk activity sites in project interviews. On St. Thomas, the market square, a bar in Smith Bay and a strip club across from St. Peter and Paul Catholic Church were selected. On St. John, a bar in Cruz Bay and the Cruz Bay Park and docking area were selected for observation. On St. Croix, several bars in downtown Frederiksted and the cemetery area in Christiansted were selected.

In each of these locations, it was clear that there was sexual activity taking place with couples leaving public areas for more private quarters. At some of the sites, there were seemingly designated areas for sexual encounters while others were for meeting people or acquiring and using drugs. One trend held across all three islands. When observations were done at different times of the day, it was evident that the same locations took on different social functions at varying hours. For example, in the market square in St. Thomas, "night people" (drug dealers, drug users, sex workers, etc.) leave in the early hours of the morning just as local vendors and merchants set up their wares in the same places that were hot spots for illicit behavior the night before. Ironically, sex workers ending their shifts in the wee hours of the morning pass by worshipers heading to early mass at the church.

The Cruz Bay area is a bustling commercial area during the day, but becomes a haven for public drug use once businesses close for the day and darkness falls. To some extent, the same is true for areas of Christiansted, but there appears to be quite a bit of illicit business going on in the Times Square area and around the cemetery even during normal business hours. This illicit activity, however, increases during the night hours. As this account suggests, risk in VI reflects a conjuncture of time, space and people. Risk is greatest at certain times (after dark), in certain places (gathering and mixing sites), and among people who regularly engage in illicit drugs/commercial sex activities.

Field team members drew maps of the 'high illicit activity areas' indicating buildings, other features, and locations where various types of risk behavior occurred. One curious finding that became evident was that on all three islands, risky activities took place in the shadow of a church. Interestingly, there appeared to be an unwritten agreement among drug dealers and sex workers that the houses of worship were 'forbidden territory.' While illicit activities took place in close proximity to churches, there appeared to be invisible boundaries that insured that activities of the spirit and those of the flesh were kept at an appropriate distance from each other. Illicit and risky HIV activities never took place directly on the church property and the immediate areas surrounding the churches were not littered or blocked. Interestingly, no such reverence is shown for the cemetery in Christiansted, where drug sales and sexual activity were commonly engaged in among the graves.

Key Informant, Rapid Intercept and Focus Group Interviews

One-on-one interview and focus group findings from the RARE assessment varied across the three islands. In response to survey questions about who in the community is most vulnerable to HIV/AIDS infection, respondents on St. Thomas ranked drug users and alcoholics as being most at risk, followed by teenagers. They also saw homosexuals at higher risk than women and sex workers, while respondents on St. Croix reversed this order. In one of the focus groups on St. Thomas, health care workers were also mentioned as a vulnerable population.

Across the three islands, night recreational sites like night clubs and bars were ranked among the riskiest sites for the transmission of HIV, although respondents on St. Thomas placed other settings, such as abandoned buildings, alleys, beaches, wooded areas, and the market area slightly higher than recreational venues. As one participant in the RARE assessment, a drug user from St. Croix, stated:

> You know, but . . . on like Prince Street, you could go around the clock, twenty-four hour, you know; they sell drink or you know people come in like I say and buy their drug. Go in a little bush and smoke . . . [leading to unprotected sex].

Public service buildings, such as schools, churches, prisons, homeless shelters, and hospitals, were ranked third, followed surprisingly by residential and illicit locations, including housing projects, commercial sex sites, and drug use areas, including shooting galleries.

As for perceived critical conditions in island communities that contribute to the spread of HIV infection, respondents across all three sites ranked lack of education about the disease and its transmission as of great importance. Respondents on St. Croix, however, viewed emotional issues such as apathy, fear, denial and social isolation as being of even greater importance; their St. Thomas counterparts cited economic conditions, including poverty, homelessness and unemployment as primary factors contributing to the spread of HIV in the VI.

With respect to AIDS risk denial, a focus group participant from St. Thomas bemoaned the fact that, "it's like that dark disease that should stay in the shadows; people are too scared of it to talk about it." Another member of this focus group related the story of a mother who became angry at an HIV specialist from St. Croix who showed her son HIV educational information. She did not want him to see or know anything about the disease. An AIDS educator who was a St. Croix focus group participant quoted a man she had tried to give information to: "I don't need that because all my women (are) clean." While he admitted to having many sexual partners, this man insisted that he knew that they were all "only with [him]." Another member of this focus group reported on a client who told a fellow service provider that he could tell if a woman was sick because if she were, he would not be able to achieve an erection.

St. John respondents cited both denial of personal risk for infection and the co-occurrence of alcohol consumption, drug use and sexual activity. These are common components of the public nightlife on St. John as well as significant promoters of HIV risk. The ready availability and use of drugs and sexual behavior, including prostitution, as well as unprotected and promiscuous sex were also seen on all of the islands as significant factors in the VI AIDS epidemic. One respondent from St. Croix commented:

> A person who needs the drug, they ain't gonna care no less that their syringe is dirty. At that moment what he wants is a syringe; it doesn't matter if it's dirty or not.

Alcohol was seen by some participants as no less risky than drug use. Thus, during a St. Thomas focus group, the following exchange occurred among participants:

> Participant One: They (people who consume alcohol) act just as crazy as the other drug users, you know.
> Participant Two: Once the alcohol gets involved, a lotta people'll go and start with the drugs . . . one thing leads to another, and [then] drugs and sex are swapped for one another.

Still, participants recognized that various factors contribute to drug abuse and risky sex beyond lack of concern or denial. Domestic violence, for example, was seen as a factor contributing to drug use and HIV risk. As one participant from St. John commented:

> [They abused women] because they're trying to escape their hurt, um, the guilt that they're, um. placed to feel because they don't really understand that it, it's really not their fault . . . they're living for escapism, so they go out and get high.

Interestingly, regarding regular commercial sex workers, a respondent on St. Thomas reported that:

> Believe it or not, the prostitutes on this island are very educated in terms of HIV/AIDS education. They're the least ones to carry it (HIV), but people that go to the prostitutes probably contracted it from someplace else.

In the focus groups, participants also discussed the importance of social class in HIV risk. Typical remarks included:

> Cause the high class people is involved in things too, you know.

> No matter how much money you have, (with) this kind of disease, if you

> Don't behave yourself, it doesn't matter who you know, where you from. . . . You don't behave yourself you be caught in the middle.

Other issues mentioned by respondents as contributors to the VI AIDS epidemic included the fact that the islands have high numbers of transients, tourists (two million per year), military personnel, and illegal aliens and a large teenage population. One participant in a St. Thomas focus group noted with regard to tourists that, "continentals [mainland residents] think they are escaping something by coming here." In the same focus group, part of the discussion focused on teenagers. Participants felt that since they grew up after the initial onslaught of the HIV/AIDS epidemic, they did not perceive the same degree of risk as the prior generation. Their tendency toward experimentation and their need for immediate gratification were also cited as causes of risky behavior among adolescents. Several participants in one of the St. Croix focus groups agreed that the prevention information for teenagers might be more effective if it came from entertainers. One participant, however, argued that materials would be more effective if they were distributed by teens trained to do peer outreach education. Another focus group participant suggested that the way to reach young people might be through visual images comprised of people who are actually infected, particularly those in later stages of the disease. There was some discussion of some of the possible pitfalls of this approach, however, including the fear that adolescents might draw the dangerous conclusion that everyone who has the disease exhibits visible physical deterioration and those who do not are disease-free.

Another suggestion from the focus groups was that youth should be included in the planning of media campaigns, rather than imposing materials on them that have been developed by adults. As one participant expressed, "We don't ask our young people anything, we tell 'em, but we never ask." It was specifically recommended that someone like Denise Stokes (a young woman who contracted HIV at the age of thirteen and was diagnosed at age sixteen when she tried to join the military) should be invited to speak to youth at a youth summit on AIDS since she could effectively communicate that adolescents are not invulnerable to the epidemic.

Cultural attitudes, such as machismo beliefs among men and having children as trophies or markers of status (something that occurs among both young women and men), were also mentioned in the focus groups. It is generally expected and largely accepted in the VI and elsewhere in the Caribbean that a man has the right to have more than one woman. This practice, in many instances, leads to a man fathering children by several different women. These 'trophy children' are viewed as a symbol of the father's masculinity, and the desire to have such markers of personal prowess is a cultural barrier to the consistent use of condoms. It is not unusual for several children fathered by the same man with different mothers, and sometimes of the same age, to attend the same school. Additionally, as one of the participants in the St. Croix focus group stated, such a man assumes (naively) that although he is having sex with many women, each of those women is only having sex with him. Regarding the issue of 'trophy children', a service provider on St. Johns remarked:

> We give out condoms, like we have birth control pills. So why do we have patients that we've seen for, . . . thirteen, fourteen years that have gotten STD after STD, have gotten pregnant, and the answer, we can't find the answer, other than, a lot of women, it seems, wants to have babies for their boyfriends. . . .

More generally, regarding the role of unequal gender relations, a respondent on St. Croix noted:

> and women, the wives, they don't know who their husband is sleeping with . . . the wife expects her husband to come back home or to go to bed and he's out foolin' around. And she might not even know. . . . Put cases on television where you see a family; the next thing you know, the wife is sick; she goes for a check-up and she has AIDS. She wasn't fooling around, but obviously somebody did. . . . I know a few cases of people [like that] who I know personally, good people. You know, you tend to think that AIDS and HIV are only for drug addicts or, you know, prostitutes; . . . hey it hits, it hits all levels.

Similarly, a service provider from St. Johns stated:

> because I do women's health 99.9% of the time, when I ask young girls about the condoms, they have the excuse that men put in their head; they say, "Oh they don't feel good. . . . And I go, how could that be? You know there's a million reasons why sex might not be feelin' good at that point, and it doesn't necessarily have to be the condom. . . . but they may have used condoms once or twice, now, (they say) Oh no, I don't like those things, I only give it to my man bareback and blah, blah, blah,' and I'm thinkin' like that's, that's man-pleasing, it's all man-pleasing with young women here.

Finally, a woman respondent on St. Thomas stated:

> I think in this community it's almost the heterosexual group that is the most vulnerable, because there's a lot of promiscuity. The least vulnerable would be those who are monogamous.

Importantly, very few respondents other than AIDS service providers were able to specifically identify existing HIV prevention services. Thus, a participant in one of the St. Thomas focus groups made the following observation:

> I don't question the effectiveness of each program. But obviously if I haven't heard of it and I've been here several months and other people here in the room haven't heard of it, they're not being too effective. . . . There are people in this room that have lived here all their lives and haven't

> heard of these programs. I mean, so, I don't think it's a matter of whether the program itself is effective, it's a matter of making sure people know about it.

Another discussion ensued in this focus group regarding why there was not more and more consistent information on AIDS in the media. It was suggested that educational campaigns are sporadic and there needs to be a consistent and continuous effort to inform the public about the changing epidemic.

The most frequently cited organizations that offer AIDS-related services were the Health Department, several HIV/AIDS programs and a number of community health clinics. Some St. John respondents, probably because of the very small population of the island (under 4,000), knew the names of individual HIV/AIDS workers more frequently than respondents on either St. Thomas or St. Croix. However, a lack of confidentiality was mentioned by several respondents when referring to the community health services on St. John. Again the small size and close familiarity of the population is a factor. This problem also was brought up during the interviews on St. Croix. One participant from St. Croix stated:

> People are afraid to go to the clinic and get a test. I wouldn't do it. I'll go to Puerto Rico; I'll go somewhere else, but I will not have a test here. . . . I work in ___ and I know what happens in clinics. . . . It's not like people are malicious or nasty or mean, it's just that because it's a small community all they have to do is tell one person, 'hey, guess who has AIDS' [and soon everyone will know].

In response to our question about the best locations to locate HIV/AIDS prevention programs, St. Croix respondents placed emphasis on discreet, accessible locations, while St. Thomas respondents stressed public and community areas, such as malls, theaters, market areas, post offices and grocery stores. St. John respondents cited schools as needing more interventions. Many of the respondents on all three islands also wanted more health services agency-based interventions. Night spots, housing projects, work places and churches all received mention as potential locations for prevention and intervention efforts. Regarding the implementation of prevention services, a female community leader on St. Thomas observed:

> People are used to turning to the government for help here, so it should be something definitely there that's available for people to get knowledge and help . . . but I also think that the kind of local counseling group should also have an area that is dedicated because many people . . . are scared of going to the government . . . but it shouldn't have any kind of moralistic tone.

A male community leader, also from St. Thomas explained:

> It's gonna take the leadership of the community in conjunction with [public and private agencies] to raise public awareness . . . from the leadership

of government, the leadership of our religious community, to be able to get the message out.

Beauty salons were identified as an under-utilized resource for AIDS prevention education. One St. Thomas focus group member affirmed:

> Every young girl in the Virgin Islands got a hairdo [that is] out of this world with six false pieces, eight false pieces, glue, and all kinds of gunk on their hair and this is an acceptable place [the salons] where they can go without being stigmatized, buy the condoms, be educated, have HIV information in there as well.

Another participant in this focus group agreed, but added that programs should be located in places where people can get information, education, support, counseling and social support all at the same time, and that the best places for this comprehensive approach are churches, community centers and schools. Another member added that information should be located in airports and cruise ship ports. When a member of the focus group reminded participants that this could have a negative impact on tourism, a primary source of income in the VI (accounting for 80% of the VI's GNP and 70% of employment), participants decided that information should be available at the post office, police stations, bars, drug stores, churches, jails and airports. One participant noted simply, "anyplace where you could buy something."

Finally, focus group participants argued for a change in AIDS education materials to better reflect the people and realities of the Virgin Islands. One focus group participant from St. Thomas complained, "all the AIDS education videos used on the islands show people from New York, California and Florida." There was general agreement in this focus group about the greater effectiveness of educational materials and programs that provide local statistics on the epidemic. Referring to a media campaign that was playing on television in the VI during the period of RARE data collection, a St. Thomas focus group participant stated the following: "Every time I watch it, I say 'Oh my God! It gets my attention every time." In this focus group, there was a great deal of stress put on the importance of making the AIDS information that is disseminated more personal and of greater relevance to the Virgin Islands.

Findings

In sum, from the diverse set of qualitative methods implemented in the Virgin Islands RARE project, project staff identified the following twelve key findings:

- Lack of AIDS information and a sense of invulnerability, combined with drug/alcohol-involvement and sexual activity among adults and youth are primary risk arenas for HIV transmission in VI.

- There are strong cultural taboos on openly identifying as a homosexual in VI. This makes it extremely difficult to identify MSM to participate in risk-reduction research and for MSMs to be reached by prevention intervention services.
- It appears that failure to use condoms is common among individuals engaged in higher risk sexual practices.
- While there is some media education on HIV/AIDS in VI, existing AIDS-prevention efforts do not adequately target those at highest risk for HIV infection.
- Churches are often found in close proximity to high-risk drug and sexual behaviors, although actual church grounds are not used for such behavior; this does not mean that the churches, however, are actively involved in AIDS prevention.
- Risk behaviors are most frequent during evening and late night periods in locations that serve other public purposes during the day.
- Alcohol consumption, not just illicit drug use, is a risk behavior for HIV. Night life sites (e.g., clubs, bars) are important sites for the combination of alcohol and unprotected sex. Beaches, crack houses and various other venues were identified as other high-risk sites.
- Lack of basic HIV transmission knowledge among sectors of the population remains an issue in VI.
- The police are often unaware of local HIV prevention services and therefore are not able to make effective referrals.
- Certain cultural practices, including the desire of men to have "trophy children" with more then one woman and the desire of women to have children for their men, create a significant risk context for HIV transmission during unprotected sex.
- Existing AIDS education videos and other materials are imported to the islands and are not culturally congruent for islanders who do not identify with the characters in the video programs.
- Beauty salons and supply houses were identified as new sites for the distribution of HIV/AIDS prevention materials.

Recommendations and Conclusions

Based on these findings, the VI RARE field team developed and submitted the following recommendations to the HIV Community Planning Groups and the Department of Health on September 28, 2001.

- Assessments should be done for HIV/AIDS risk among youth in the VI, from the middle teens to the late twenties.

- MSMs, especially MSMs who also have sex with women, should be a high priority for assessment and HIV/AIDS prevention efforts in the VI.
- Community agencies providing services should expand their HIV/prevention and referral efforts both to the general population and to high risk target groups.
- Churches are uniquely positioned (geographically) for targeted prevention and should be recruited for expanded involvement in prevention efforts.
- Prevention efforts must be pushed beyond the 9–5 daytime business time zone to include late night prevention efforts in high-risk locations.

These recommendations, and the data and findings of the VI RARE project have been incorporated by the HIV Community Planning Group into the development of its subsequent comprehensive plans. Prior to the year 2000 there was hardly any local data available for the HIV-prevention community planning effort. Project RARE helped to fill a notable and strongly felt gap in the development of prevention that was grounded in local realities and knowledge on risk behaviors, attitudes and locations. Additionally, by closely linking data collection and qualitative methodology with intervention, Project RARE helped to demonstrate the value of using qualitative research as a community-based tool in the fight against AIDS. Statistics on AIDS in the Virgin Islands make clear; even in 'paradise,' there is a critical need for resources to confront an ongoing epidemic that already has taken a painful toll in human life and suffering.

References

Castro, Arachu, Farmer, P. (2004) Pearls of the Antilles? Public Health in Haiti and Cuba. In Arachu Castro and Merrill Singer, eds. *Unhealthy Health Policy: A Critical Anthropological Examination.* (pp. 3–28). Walnut Creek, CA: Altamira.

Needle, R., Trotter, R., II, Singer, M., et al. (2003) "Rapid Assessment of the HIV/AIDS Crisis in Racial and Ethnic Minority Communities: An Approach for Timely Community Interventions." *American Journal of Public Health* 93 (6): 970–979.

Trotter, R., II, Needle, R., Goosby, E., et al. (2001) "A Methodological Model for Rapid Assessment, Response, and Evaluation: The RARE Program in Public Health." *Field Methods* 13 (2): 137–159.

Virgin Islands HIV Community Planning Group (2000) *The United States Virgin Islands HIV Prevention Comprehensive Plan.* U.S. Virgin Islands: Virgin Islands Department of Health.

Chapter 11

The RARE Experience in Miami

Louis Herns Marcelin
Bryan Page

In Miami-Dade, as elsewhere in the United States, HIV and AIDS disproportionately affect minority populations, especially those of African descent. This is partly due to the fact that AIDS in the U.S. has taken a new direction over the last ten years, as the dissemination of highly active anti-retroviral therapy (HAART) has broadened, reducing the contribution to the incidence of new HIV infections the segment of the U.S. population that enjoys access to adequate health care (CDC 2004). White non-Hispanic men who have sex with men still dominate the cumulative prevalence statistics on AIDS in the U.S., but ethnic minority populations have increased their rates of new cases (CDC 2001, 2004), displaying rates of new HIV infection many times those of other major populations. Adolescent and adult black men, for example, had an estimated rate of new infections of 108 per 100,000 in 2002. This rate was almost nine times higher than that of adolescent and adult white men (12.3 per 100,000). The differential between black females' rate and that of white females is even more striking: 48.6 per 100,000 versus 2.1 per 100,000—more than twenty fold. Young people (under age 25) in ethnic minority populations have increased their numbers of new cases relative to the white populations and therefore increased cumulative prevalence (CDC 2001, 2004; Rosenberg, Biggar, and Goedert 1994).

In the year 2000, more blacks were reported with AIDS and estimated to be living with AIDS, than any other racial or ethnic group in the U.S. (CDC 2001). In 1999, Florida ranked third of all states with HIV/AIDS as cause of death for people of ages 25–44 and first for all black males and females of the same age group. Although they represent approximately 13.9% of the Florida population (Census 2000), people of African descent now account for 46% of the 79,155 AIDS cases reported through December 2000 and 59% of the 19,149 HIV cases reported between 1997 and December 2000 (Florida Department of Health

Health 2001). This compares to 54% of new HIV infections and 47% of new AIDS cases in the U.S. (CDC 2001). Select seroprevalence studies among at risk populations provide evidence that the HIV/AIDS epidemic is increasingly concentrated in low-income communities with predominantly Black populations. As in other settings in the U.S., in Miami-Dade, epidemiological reports, however, are formulated within a demographic frame that lumps every Black individual in the same generic category "Black or African American." Aggregate epidemiological data on Blacks say very little about the trend of HIV infection among immigrant Black populations and obscure the increasing diversity of the Black communities, such as Bahamians, Haitians, Jamaicans and other Caribbean immigrants. The Rapid Assessment Response and Evaluation conducted in Miami-Dade between September 1999 and March 2000 has to be placed within this larger background.

In response to the initiative announced by the Department of Health and Human Services/Office of HIV/AIDS Policy (DHHS/OHAP), the office of the Mayor made a formal request for the technical assistance offered by the Department. The Rapid Assessment process was overseen by a community working group (CWG) which, at the end of the process, took the major recommendations and transformed them into action steps to be implemented in Miami-Dade.

Based on the Miami-Dade's Department of Health HIV and AIDS prevalence data, the Community Advisory Committee recommended that the team should focus on four zip codes: 33127, 33136, 33147, and 33150. These geographical areas constitute the most segregated areas of Miami-Dade, where marginalized populations have not been in a position to combat endemic social ills, such as violence, poor access to services and poverty. At the time of the RARE implementation in Miami-Dade, there were no epidemiological data available on specific populations, such as Haitian immigrants and other Caribbean Blacks. Moreover, as it is the case for the rest of the country, current infrastructure for planning and implementation of programs relies heavily on geo-epidemiological data from federal and state surveillance systems. In this sense, the use of zip-code data as means to assess differential geographical distribution of HIV and AIDS cases in Miami-Dade has been critical to RARE.

Methods

The field team gathered five kinds of data: Team members spent scores of person-hours in each of the chosen sites watching the human activity, while maintaining a focus on how drug use and sexual behavior combine to produce risk of HIV infection.

1. Field-notes: Staff spent a great deal of time writing and/or tape recording notes on what they saw in the places where sex is exchanged for drugs or money. These notes took nothing for granted.

2. Informal interviews—While they were observing, the team members

necessarily had to come into contact with people in those locales, explaining what they were doing and asking questions about the conditions in the neighborhood. Accounts of these informal interviews became part of the observers' field notes, quoting conversations verbatim at times, and paraphrasing others.

3. Intensive interviews with individuals—Some people found in the street were so knowledgeable and articulate that it was worthwhile to interview them formally. Field assessors set up appointments with individuals identified in this way for the purpose of conducting a tape-recorded interview. In these interviews, field interviewers encouraged the person to speak freely on the topics of interest. As with the field notes, the tape recordings of these conversations were transcribed into electronic files for later analysis.

4. Focus groups--Knowledgeable people in the community contributed additional insights when they talked in groups that focused on topics of particular interest. These focus groups consisted of people selected by the field workers to discuss the same issues discussed in the individual interviews. The field team conducted at least one focus group in each of the chosen sites. These groups consisted primarily of people at risk who spoke about the nature of HIV risk in their own neighborhoods

5. Mapping risk behavior—Because the zones chosen for study were large, the research team used maps of these zones to pinpoint specific places in which we observed behavior related to risk.

Data Analysis

Weekly meetings—Every Tuesday between October 1 and December 14, the team met to discuss the week's activities and findings. Specific observations and interviews revealed notable conditions in need of intervention, such as the routine arrest by police of men carrying condoms in the Little Havana stroll. We discussed the implications of this information in terms of what more we needed to find out about the conditions, who was most affected, and what needed to be done to remedy the situation. Proceedings of these meetings guided further inquiry and helped the coordinators to assess the progress of efforts in the various sites for assessment. Ultimately, the weekly meetings' outcomes guided the analysis of the collected data.

Electronic files—The vast majority of the team's data consisted of verbal descriptions and conversations. Once we had recorded these words in word processing files, we could use search utilities in text management software to find passages and phrases that described specific aspects of the behavior observed in risk sites and the words of participants that interpreted this action. For example, we looked through all of the field notes to find places where the observer described how people who wanted to exchange sex or money for drugs found each other. Using key words, such as "encounter," "meet," and "cruise," we found parts of the field notes that described those actions. We also looked through the interviews and focus groups to find the places in which participants spoke about these actions. We then arrayed these passages to develop an understanding of how people link up with each other in the risk locales. We used this procedure repeatedly in order to develop the concept of "place" that appears in the report.

Findings

The combined experience of intensive field observations, interviews, focus groups, and regular meetings to process the week's data enabled the investigators to structure the nature of risk in the targeted neighborhoods according to three basic concepts: people, place, and time. The presentations that follow use that structure in delineating risk of infection by the HIV as we found it in each of these neighborhoods.

How Does Risk Happen?

Risk happens when drugs and sex keep company, and the targeted communities each presented the field researchers with different profiles regarding people, place, and time. When the assessment teams observed activities in the chosen zones and interviewed the people about what kinds of risk occurred there, they repeatedly heard and saw that the highest risk of exposure to HIV happens in settings where sex is exchanged for drugs or money. These exchanges took place between different people for different reasons in the sites observed by the field team. Below (Table 11.1) is an outline of interactions between people, place, and time (see also Needle et. al. 2003).

Table 11.1: Mixing patterns between people place and time

Neighborhoods	People	Place	Time	Mobility
Little Haiti	Sex for money (mostly young female)	*Makrel* (in Haitian Creole stands for transit house); Parks; Empty lots	Late night (mostly on weekends); Weekdays between 8 p.m. and midnight	Clients commute in for sex (from Broward County and South of Miami-Dade)
Edison Transitional	Sex for drugs and money; Injection Drug Users (heroin and crack)	Get-off houses (crack houses); Park; Abandoned buildings	24 hours in get-off houses; Sunset to sunrise in abandoned buildings; 9 p.m.-3 a.m. in Parks	Sex workers and clients commuting in for sex and drugs
Liberty City	Sex for drugs (sex workers, MSM and young addicts)	Get-off houses; Park; Abandoned buildings	24 hours in crack houses Sunset to sunrise in abandoned buildings	Sex workers and clients commuting in for sex and drugs
Little Havana	Sex for drugs (mostly MSM) and money; Injection Drug Users (heroin and crack)	Adult bookstores; Empty lots (in car); Abandoned buildings	Late afternoon; Late night (mostly on weekends) in empty lots	Local customers; Some MSM commute for sex and drugs

The relationship between sex and drug use as motivators for risk varied in two ways among the zones chosen for study: either drugs drove the sex, or sex drove the drugs. In the former case, sex workers made sex available because they needed to obtain more drugs. In the latter case, clientele of sex workers converged on certain places because they could find people willing to accept cash in return for sexual service. This latter kind of sex worker could opt to buy drugs after the cash transaction, but the former always moved as quickly as possible to obtaining drugs. The descriptions presented below begin by characterizing sex-for-money versus sex-for-drugs transactions (see Table 2 above).

Little Haiti

Sex Drives Drugs: Risk of sexual exposure to HIV takes several forms in Little Haiti, but the exchange of sex for money appears to have primary importance in the places where risk occurs. Customers from other parts of South Florida, as far north as West Palm Beach and as far south as the Keys, commute to Little Haiti in order to seek sexual adventures and fantasies with young, poor Haitians. Availability of drugs to these sex workers appears secondary to the workers' obtaining money for sex. The sex transactions usually happen in what the locals call "*makrel*," which refers to a house of prostitution. These *makrel* are relatively invisible for outsiders who are not part of the sex networks. They are regular houses with no identifier or sign that may stand apart from other houses in the neighborhood. In one zip code alone, our research team identified seven highly frequented *makrel* with dense networks of clients. The pattern 'sex-for-money-money-for-drugs' contrasts with the patterns found in the other focal areas of assessment.

Person—Females fourteen to thirty years old dominated the sex trade. Clients of sex workers ranged into the sixties, but most were in their thirties and forties. Many of the clients came from distant sites, seeking to play out sexual fantasies with young sex workers in Little Haiti.

Edison Transitional

Drugs Drive Sex: In this neighborhood where African American and Haitian populations come together, the sex trade has come to operate on the assumption that drug addicts and sex workers use sex to obtain drugs. Clients of these workers can utilize either money or drugs to manipulate the sex workers' behavior. Because the drugs of choice among the sex workers, especially crack and, to a lesser extent, heroin, have a strong association with dependence and obsessive use, the clients assume that sex workers in this zone are desperate for drugs. Some clients even prefer to have drugs to offer sex workers directly, because the latter's desperation makes possible extreme manipulation of their behavior in playing out the client's fantasies of dominance and control. In this setting, clients can demand even the riskiest sexual behaviors of the sex worker and find someone willing to gratify their desires.

Place and Time—Park is a category of site where risk takes place in the transitional neighborhood, again, with restrictions on time. Risk activities, although not exclusively taking place at night, tended to happen in the park after sunset. During the day, the park had many uses besides risky ones, but after sunset, especially late at night, it became a venue for finding sex partners and using drugs. Crack houses also operate in the Edison area, and the team has observed both un-staffed and staffed crack houses there. These places operate around the clock, but their most intense activity occurs at night.

Person—Males and females fourteen and older participated in the combined risks of sex and drugs at this site. Risk behavior in these contexts consisted of both men and women selling sex (more men than women) and primarily men buying sex or exchanging drugs for it. Although the youngest participants were in their teens, people over thirty predominated in this area.

Liberty City

Drugs Drive Sex: Again, the assumption that drug addicts and sex workers are desperate to obtain drugs dominates the combination of drugs with sex. Drug addicts and sex workers who primarily care about obtaining their next "hit" find themselves constantly in risky situations. Clients may actually prefer to have a "hit" on their persons in order to find a willing sex worker quickly. Clientele of sex workers also commute into Liberty City, the traditional home of African Americans in Dade County, but much of the sex trade originates within the neighborhood.

Place and Time—Park also operates in Liberty City on a system in which people use the place for one purpose during the day and another at night. After midnight, men who have sex with men seek partners or a place in which to bring a partner from elsewhere. Those desiring drugs can also find them at these hours in the park. Bus stops provide a place where men who have sex with men can make contacts with other men while appearing to wait for the bus. People sitting at the bus stop make contacts with potential sex partners or simply wait for a bus, but the onlooker has few hints as to which of the two purposes is given to a bench full of men at the time of observation. A library offers a place for rest and for seeking sexual partners, where sex acts may take place in the rest rooms or secluded corners. Liberty City has crack houses in which drug use and sexual risk take place, and they operate around the clock, but most intensively between sunset and sunrise.

Person—Males and females fourteen and older combined sexual behavior and drug use in a complex of HIV risk. As in Edison, both sexes participated in sex trade, but women predominated as sellers of sex. Men predominated as buyers, and people over thirty years old were the principal actors in this scene.

East Little Havana

Drugs Drive Sex: As in Liberty City and Edison, the observed risk behavior began with the desire of the drug addicts and sex workers to obtain drugs, specifically crack cocaine, but these workers were predominantly male. Not only did the clientele of these sex workers commute into the neighborhood, but some of the sex workers commuted as well, from as far away as Broward County. The desire for crack cocaine made the sex workers interviewed and observed in Little Havana engage in very risky behavior. The clients seldom offered drugs directly, but the sex workers quickly converted their fees into crack cocaine.

Place and Time—Crack house, in the team's observations, was an abandoned building convenient to the observed sex worker's stroll. It had no staff, and operated around the clock, but most intensively at night. In keeping with the fluid nature of the sex workers' strolls, the clients' cars afforded a place where sexual risk behavior could occur. Once the sex worker boarded the car, the driver could choose a secluded place in which to purchase sex acts. Adult bookstores also presented opportunities for sexual encounters in back rooms. These encounters could take the form of either spontaneous liaisons or paid transactions. The bookstores' most intensive activity took place in the late afternoon and early evening.

Person—Males and females both took part in sexual risk in this assessed area, but very few females. Ages of both sex workers and clients ranged between twenty and forty years old.

Recommendations

Each of the following recommendations emanates from some aspect of the field work summarized above. In some cases, the recommendations resulted from specific observations made in the targeted zones. In others, interviews with local participants at risk or people who have worked to reduce risk in certain areas. Each recommendation will be preceded by a brief statement on how we derived it from the RARE process.

Outreach Presence—The field team encountered no risk reduction outreach activities in any of the zones studied although some were known to operate in the area. The field team tended to enter the areas when risk was taking place, while the known outreach efforts took place 9 p.m. to 5 p.m. on weekdays.

> Recommendation 1: Outreach agents must establish a presence at the place when people have risky sex, especially sex closely related to drug use.

The venues described above in the section on place, seldom if ever have an outreach presence advocating prevention of HIV and encouraging use of care facilities. Either roaming outreach specialists or outreach satellite offices need to operate or to be located in or near sex workers' strolls, districts known to have crack houses, and parks where risky behavior takes place.

Recommendation 2: Outreach agents need to be available at hours when clientele are receptive to services and education.

Sex worker strolls are busiest between 10:00 p.m. and 4:00 a.m., and crack houses and their environs are most active between sunset and sunup. Yet most services and outreach operate during regular daylight business hours. Even if more service providers and outreach efforts were located near the points of highest activity, they might attract no clientele because they were not operating when the clientele is most active and potentially receptive.

Recommendation 3: Offer the services in places identified with generic health concerns, not with AIDS only.

This is important because the clientele wants to avoid stigma attached to AIDS-only venues and services: make those venues and services "health generic." We base this recommendation primarily on interviews with persons at risk. Strategies to accomplish the removal of stigma would begin with training health workers who deliver outreach on other health issues to work the areas identified in this assessment and to deliver AIDS-related outreach. Whether they worked directly on the street, out of a store-front office, or out of a generic health van, these workers would not carry the same stigma as AIDS-only workers carry.

Recommendation 4: Use existing health van services to enhance outreach by cross-training van staff in AIDS.

This recommendation ties together recommendations 1–3. Community workers familiar with the zones under study made the specific recommendation to cross-train workers on existing health vans and to have them target the assessed areas at times of greatest activity.

Recommendation 5: Conduct micro-interventions in risk locales, such as condom distribution and HIV testing on strolls.

Certain kinds of on-the-spot interventions suggested themselves to the field teams as they observed some of the assessed zones. They included the distribution of condoms to people engaged in sex trade (with reservations described in later recommendations) and on-site HIV testing. We refer to these as micro-interventions. The people participating in these risk locales told the field team

Recommendation 6: Fund innovative health services vehicles, such as vans, that place outreach at risk locales, and/or permanent centers for prevention and intervention.

As they currently operate, the health vans do not really serve the places assessed in this exercise, nor do any of the stationary centers in the targeted neighborhoods. We therefore recommend funding innovative vehicles for delivering the kinds of intervention that these sites need. Mobile vans that offer generic health aid and distribute prevention materials, or new street-side offices open at strategic times for reaching the clientele, exemplify this approach to improving the reach of intervention into the assessed areas.

Recommendation 7: Recruit natural leaders in risk sites to participate in interventions.

Some people who live in or very close to the places where risk occurs have expressed their willingness to help. We strongly suggest that people like that in each of the affected communities receive the necessary training and some modest material support toward helping to protect their neighbors from risk of HIV infection. One such individual speaks in the following interview:

> Interviewer: How do you call the house?
> Respondent: It is my house. I don't call it no kinda house or nothing like that, you know. Everybody say my name. I'm (name), you know what I'm saying? Let's go by (name) house, you know, and just sit in thare and I look out for people and try to help them out, you know, what I'm sayin'? They don't have no place to go. I won't put nobody on the street if I have a place to sleep. It ain't much, but grab a spot here and there, you know.
> Int: So basically you offer them, you know, places for them to wash up.
> Resp: To wash up and buy them clothes, and stuff from the warehouse and I give them. . . .
> Give them clothes and stuff. Like it is starting to get cold now, you know. I've been trying to get jackets and coats and stuff like that, too.

Clearly, this person has spontaneously tried to help participants in the zone of intensive risk in his own way. With some training and encouragement, his intervention could have an impact on the well-being of his clientele in ways that help to prevent AIDS.

Hours of HIV-related agencies—In the community wide focus group and in our interviews with potential clientele, it became clear that agencies that maintained standard business hours were not even open when people engaged in serious risk were circulating in the community. We made the following recommendation as in answer to that expressed discrepancy.

Recommendation 8: Expand or re-structure service hours in existing agencies.

People at risk cannot come to agencies that are only open during the business day, especially if they are not near where they live. We suggest times for remaining open as follows: 5:00 to 8:00 p.m. for working people; 10:00 p.m. to 2:00 a.m. for sex workers and people with drug-related risk.

Access to Treatment for Drug Abuse—Inevitably, when field research teams come into contact with active drug users, they will hear about the users' desire to seek treatment and the unavailability of treatment slots. This recommendation emanates from the field team's experiences hearing this kind of complaint.

Recommendation 9: Improve access to treatment for drug abuse.

If coupled with better outreach, improved (on-demand) access to treatment can engage people at risk before they change their minds. Many of the informal interviewees, formal interviewees, and participants in focus groups indicated that they would be willing to go into treatment for drug abuse if they had better access. Their difficulties with access included lack of available slots when they presented, being "tested" by the clinicians to make sure they would stick, and no treatment facilities near where they lived. Given the clear connection between intensive drug use and intensive sexual risk of HIV in this assessment, recommendation three was inevitable.

Poster Placement—Particularly in a bookstore venue in Little Havana, but also in bars in various zones, the field team observed high volume of client traffic but not much coverage of key wall space with AIDS preventive posters. We therefore made the following recommendation based on these observations.

Recommendation 10: Place posters in key places.

Public places in which risk begins and/or occurs seldom have basic warning messages about condom use and safer sex. Bars, restrooms in bars, adult bookstores, and bus stations should be required though a bi-county ordinance to have such posters on prominent display.

Education of Police—Observed and reported comportment of police in all of the zones under study fell short of what we would consider optimal handling of HIV-related behavior. We made the next based on this experience.

Recommendation 11: Police need education on strategies for reducing risk among people at risk, especially regarding condom use.

Sex workers reported to members of the field team that police were profiling individuals as sex workers if they had condoms on their persons. Consequently, the sex workers reported that they were unwilling to carry condoms for fear of arrest. We recommend that police abolish policies of profiling people as sex workers on the basis of possession of condoms. Sex workers are the last people we want to be afraid to carry condoms.

Condom placement in risk locales—We repeatedly found sex workers with no access to any condoms in the midst of very high sex trade traffic. The investigators recommended that condoms be made available, either by outreach personnel or dispensing machines near risk sites.

Recommendation 12: Place condoms in risk locales.

Sex workers reported to the assessment team that when on the job, they were unwilling to stop work in order to obtain condoms. Sex workers and heavy drug users stay so busy getting tricks and drugs that they don't want to leave to get condoms. Places where people trick and combine sex with drugs should have dispensers of condoms or some other way of delivering them just at the time the user needs them. Dispensing of condoms at the times and in the places where sex workers operate will increase the proportion of protected sexual contacts in the assessed areas.

AIDS education for people who patronize sex workers—The field team had some contact with patrons of risk locales, and informal conversations with them revealed their ignorance about basic principles of HIV contagion. We therefore recommended a course for "johns."

Recommendation 13: Educate "johns" in HIV/AIDS risk and prevention.

In all of the assessed areas, the interviewees and observations showed that much of the sex workers' risky behaviors could be traced to the demands of the clients, or "johns." Because they are the ones who have the money and who dictate how the trick goes, clients of sex workers need to receive education on prevention of HIV. We therefore recommend that, when arrested for solicitation, johns should be required to get education on HIV (i.e., "104," the designation of the standard course on AIDS required of county health workers).

Dissemination of audio media on AIDS—This recommendation did not emanate so much from the field work as from the investigators' previous experience in attempting to distribute AIDS educational materials. Illiteracy is widespread among Haitians in Miami/Dade County, and audio presentations of AIDS education can succeed in reaching some of that population.

Recommendation 14: Distribute and publicly play audio tapes containing messages on prevention of AIDS.

Especially in the Haitian community, the tradition of sending and receiving audio cassettes has strong potential as a vehicle for disseminating Public Service Announcements. These cassettes can be recorded with messages about AIDS and duplicated for wide distribution, or they can be played on Haitian radio programs or over loudspeakers at strategic points in the community.

and duplicated for wide distribution, or they can be played on Haitian radio programs or over loudspeakers at strategic points in the community.

Risk due to injection of drugs—Interviews with IDUs, observation of risk behavior, and focus groups all pointed out low availability of clean needle/syringe sets (N/S) in the zones under study. Presentation of the recommendation to governmental authorities supported advocacy of needle exchanges (Florida maintains paraphernalia laws that forbid it).

Recommendation 15: Start needle exchanges in high-risk areas at night.

Availability of needle/syringe sets (N/S) was noticeably low in the zones where the assessment team worked. As this condition leads to re-use of contaminated N/S, we recommend improvement of availability of N/S. Cleansing solution (bleach kits), clean cookers and water, although available, need to be distributed in time and on-site where people are using drugs intravenously. These materials were usually not present in the sites where the teams conducted observations.

Evidence compiled by three different federal blue-ribbon panels since 1997 have summarized the impact of needle exchanges as follows:

- They reduce the frequency of drug use by injection among program participants.
- They do not increase the number of new initiates to injection drug use.
- They reduce the reuse and "sharing" of blood-contaminated injection equipment.
- They facilitate entry into drug treatment.
- They do not result in increased numbers of discarded syringes.
- They prevent the transmission of HIV.

Based on our own observations and the findings of these blue-ribbon panels, we recommend that Dade County consider implementation of needle exchange programs.

Continue rapid assessment—This recommendation comes in recognition of how much useful information and insight that impact policy can be had from this technique for assessing community health problems.

Recommendation 16: Continue and extend the process of rapid assessment.

The participants in this training and assessment exercise found it both rewarding and absorbing. Through it, we came to recognize that, although we had extensive experience in affected communities, the RARE techniques enabled us to discover aspects of HIV in Miami/Dade County that we would not otherwise have found out. We also came to realize how much more we need to discover the county make available resources to train a group of assessment specialists to identify new areas of acute need. We also recommend that the county hire a full-time ethno-epidemiologist to advise and supervise rapid assessments here. Finally, we recommend that the county incorporate ongoing rapid assessment into its master plan and the Community Prevention Plan.

Conclusion and Outcome

Since the RARE experience in Miami in 2000, the local health department has incorporated the methodology in its own outreach strategy. During the last two years, at least two rapid assessments have been implemented in other deprived and at-risk neighborhoods. However, as funding for HIV/AIDS prevention is declining, community members where RARE has been originally implemented are still holding questions regarding the future of RARE. Most of the recommendations that could have been implemented in the neighborhoods studied have been placed on hold because of lack of funding, despite the demonstrated commitment of the local health department to effective prevention. Moreover, most RARE recommendations carried with them the inherent difficulty to coordinate different agencies in implementing them. Indeed, how the information collected was understood by policy makers and local authorities is not clear. One of the former field team members put it this way: "I guess the major challenge for RARE is political will. We have got to get those people that are in those places where they make decisions to hear us. This seems not to happen in the near future." But still, one can capitalize on the positive impact of RARE in Miami-Dade.

The local health department is incorporating the RARE strategy and findings into its own intervention project. According to a local health official, the number of people educated has increased and the number of people tested has also increased. The local health department has modified its outreach practices in terms of repositioning the presence of outreach workers in space and time. The outreach has definitely had some effect. Moreover, an increasing number of contractors have changed their schedules to accommodate the nighttime outreach instead of daytime outreach when a lot of people are at work.

References

CDC (1990). *HIV AIDS Surveillance Report*. Atlanta: Centers for Disease Control and Prevention.

CDC (2000). *HIV AIDS Surveillance Report Supplement*. Atlanta: Centers for Disease Control and Prevention

CDC (2001). *Young People at Risk: HIV and AIDS among America's Youth*. Atlanta: Centers for Disease Control and Prevention.

CDC (2001). *Young People at Risk: HIV and AIDS among America's Youth.* Atlanta: Centers for Disease Control and Prevention.

CDC (2004). *HIV AIDS Surveillance Report.* Atlanta: Centers for Disease Control and Prevention.

Needle R.H., Trotter, R.T., II, Goosby, E., et al. (1999). *Crisis Response Teams and Communities Combat HIV/AIDS in Racial and Ethnic Minority Populations: A Guide for Conducting Community-Based Rapid Assessment, Rapid Response, and Evaluation.* Washington, D.C.: U.S. Dept of Health and Human Services, Office of HIV/AIDS Policy.

Needle R.H., Trotter, R.T., II, Goosby E. (2000) "Methodologically Sound Rapid Assessment and Response: Providing Timely Data for Policy Development on Drug Use Interventions." *Int J Drug Policy.* 11: 19–23.

Needle, R.H., Trotter, R.T., II, Singer, M. (2003) "Rapid Assessment of the HIV/AIDS Crisis in Racial and Ethnic Minority Communities: An Approach for Timely Community Interventions." *American Journal of Public Health* 93 (6): 970–980.

Singer M. (1999). Studying hidden and hard-to-research populations. In Schensul, J.J., LeCompte, M.D., Trotter, R.T. II, et al. (eds.) *Mapping Networks, Spatial Data, and Hidden Populations.* (pp. 1–36) The Ethnographer's Toolkit, Vol. 4. Walnut Creek, Calif: Altamira Press.

Trotter, R.T., II, Needle, R.H., Goosby, E. et al. (2001) "A Methodological Model for Rapid Assessment, Response, and Evaluation: the RARE Program in Public Health." *Field Methods.* 13 (2): 137–159.

Trotter, II, R.T., Needle, R.H. (1999) *Crisis Response Teams and Communities Combat HIV/AIDS in Racial and Ethnic Minority Populations: Rapid Assessment, Rapid Response, and Evaluation Field Assessment Training Workbook.* Washington: U.S. Dept of Health and Human Services, Office of HIV/AIDS Policy.

Chapter 12

Twilight's Last Gleaning: Rapid Assessment of Late Night HIV Risk in Hartford, CT

Merrill Singer
Julie Eiserman

At the Edge of the Epicenter: Life and AIDS in Hartford

Hartford, Connecticut, an old American city that for non-residents brings to mind deep-hued New England foliage, the industrial Yankee heartland, and the hub of the insurance industry is, as well, the fourth poorest moderate-size city in the country. While the state of Connecticut is populated by residents who have higher incomes, lower unemployment rates, and more years of education than the nation as a whole, the same is not true of its capitol, Hartford. Of the fourteen poorest cities in the U.S., Hartford was one of only four that saw an increase in the rate of poverty between 1990 and 2000 (Connecticut Department of Health 2002); the percentage of people living below the federal poverty line in Hartford increased from 3.1% to 30.6% of the city's total population during this period. The average per capita income in Hartford is $13,428, the lowest of any city in the state (Connecticut Department of Health 2003).

With such a high concentration of poverty, social conditions in Hartford are tenuous: 58% of families with children are headed by a single female; 39% of adults lack a high school degree; and unemployment is three times that for the state (Trinity College 2001). Moreover, 22% of all births in Hartford in 2000 were to teenage mothers (compared to 14% across the 50 U.S. cities with the highest teen birth rates). In Hartford, more teenage girls give birth than graduate from high school (Trinity College 2001). During 1999, the rate of the STI (sexually transmitted infection), chlamydia, in Hartford was more than double the national rate and four times the rate of the state of Connecticut (Hartford Courant 2001). Across the ten indicators used by the Annie E. Casey Foundation as an interlocked set of factors that effectively measure child wellbeing (i.e., rates of low birth weight, infant mortality, child death, teen death, teen birth, school dropout, parental unemployment, teens not working or going to school, child poverty, single parent households, and lack of employment opportunities), Hartford compares poorly to other cities in the nation (Trinity College 2001). Finally, there is the issue of ethnic disparities. Of the children born in Hartford in 2000, 48% were Latino, and 42% were African American (Annie E. Casey Foundation 2003). In addition to poverty, Hartford residents suffer ethnic/racial discrimination, wealthier cities in Connecticut which are populated by mostly whites resist efforts to use state dollars to solve the capital's socio-economic woes.

All of these factors put Hartford at high risk for poor health indicators, given existing national patterns of ethnic differences in health status (Smedley, Stith and Nelson 2003). In reference to the AIDS epidemic, Hartford forms part of the hinterland of the New York/New Jersey megalopolis, an epicenter of the national and international AIDS epidemic. Consequently, Connecticut ranks 9th in its rate of AIDS cases per 100,000 population nationally, and within the state of Connecticut, the city with the most reported cases of AIDS is Hartford, with 2,719 total cases (Connecticut Department of Health 2003). Sixty-three percent of people living with AIDS (PLWAs) in Hartford are injection drug users (IDUs); 16% are non-IDUs with heterosexual risk; and 11% are non-IDU men who have sex with men (MSM). Forty-eight percent of PLWAs in Hartford are Latino, while 38% are black. Twenty-nine percent of all PLWAs in Hartford are women.

These statistics qualified Hartford as a site for the national RARE initiative. The RARE Hartford Project was implemented through the Hispanic Health Council, a community-based research, direct service and advocacy agency that began community education on AIDS in 1983 and public health research on AIDS in 1988. This chapter describes the RARE Hartford Project, key project findings, and the impact of the project on AIDS and related work in the city.

Methodology

The RARE Hartford Project was guided by a Community Advisory Working Group (CAWG) comprised of the City Health Director, the local Ryan White Title 1 Director, and representatives of community-based organizations, AIDS service organizations, and drug treatment agencies. This group selected late night risk in the north and south ends of the city as their topic of interest to be investigated using RARE rapid assessment procedures (Needle et al. 2003; Singer 200;, Trotter. et al. 2001). The project team was assembled in July of 2003 and, following training by the project director and coordinator, began conducting ethnographic observation at night on July 31, 2003.

The research began with a free listing exercise in which all team members listed possible sites of late-night sex- and drug-related risk in Hartford. Once the list was completed, sites were prioritized in terms of expected levels of risk activity. Two-person teams were assigned particular sites to visit and observe after 11 p.m. on designated nights of the week. Initially, field team members, individuals with a range of backgrounds in AIDS outreach, community service, and research, took short notes at the site or in their cars based on their observations. Once they left the field, they wrote or typed more detailed versions of their notes, which they turned in at the weekly project meetings. The field team also was asked to draw basic maps of the high-risk locations that they visited and label streets, businesses, and specific sites of high-risk activities.

The field team began conducting intercept surveys with individuals at observed sites on August 11, 2003. Field team members stopped individuals at the identified sites and asked them if they would be willing to complete a short survey. The questions asked in these brief street intercept survey interviews addressed: 1) personal socio-demographic characteristics; 2) knowledge of local sites that have a high degree of risk behaviors; 3) knowledge of late-night, high risk groups in Hartford; 4) types of late night, high-risk behaviors in Hartford; 5) exposure to HIV prevention information; and 6) perception of HIV/AIDS related needs in Hartford. The surveys lasted approximately ten minutes. After leaving the field site, field team members wrote expanded accounts of participants' answers based on notes taken during the interviews. The participants did not receive a financial incentive for participation, but the field team did give out free condoms while conducting fieldwork at the sites. The field team completed sixty-seven street intercept surveys, seven surveys beyond the goal. The survey results were reviewed and used for structuring questions on other study instruments.

The field team began conducting in-depth interviews in mid-August with individuals who fell into at least one of four late-night behavioral groups: drug users of any type of drugs (DU), drug sellers (DS), men who have sex with men (MSM), and commercial sex workers (SW). Non-injecting drug users were included because they have far higher than average levels of HIV infection in Hartford, may have been or may become IDUs over time, and because of the field team's knowledge that some drug users exchange sex for drugs or money and/or engage in risky sex under the influence of drugs. Drug sellers were included because of the field team's knowledge that some drug sellers are also drug users and/or exchange drugs for sex with their customers. In order to determine risk factors, the participants were also asked whether or not they had multiple sex partners or ever paid for sex. The field team completed thirty-one in-depth interviews.

Some of the participants in the in-depth interviews had completed surveys first, and proved to be informative individuals; others were recruited through conversations at the target sites. Of those, some were given business cards and asked to contact the field coordinator to make an appointment for an interview at the Hispanic Health Council. Others were interviewed on the spot at the site. A third group of interviewees was referred by other participants, who were recruited during the night and had completed interviews. For example, the initial interviews were conducted with members of one social network of Latino sex workers/drug users. The first interviewee was recruited by members of the field team through night outreach. She was a self-identified lesbian Latina commercial sex worker who used crack and heroin and had sex for money or drugs with men during the night. During the interview, she explained that she had many acquaintances and friends, both male and female, who also did commercial sex work at night for money to buy drugs. Upon the field coordinator's request, she referred some of these individuals to the project to complete the interview. The in-depth interview took between forty-five minutes and one and a half hours to complete, and all of these interviews were audio-taped. Participants were paid an incentive of $20.

The field team also conducted focus groups with community members who had experience with or knowledge of late-night risk activities in Hartford. Participants for the focus groups were also either recruited during late-night fieldwork or through other participants in the study. The project team had a goal of conducting at least three focus groups, but was able to conduct five focus groups with thirty-one community members. Each focus group was conducted with individuals who shared a common risk category. The number of participants in the focus group varied between five and ten members.

Most focus groups were conducted at the Hispanic Health Council. Two focus groups, with participants who identified themselves as drug sellers, were conducted in the homes of participants in order to make them feel more comfortable. The focus groups took between one and two hours to complete and were audio-taped. These participants were also paid $20 for their time. The field team completed the late-night ethnographic fieldwork on September 20, 2003, when recruitment for the targeted number of intercept surveys, in-depth interviews, and focus groups with community members was complete.

Participants in both the in-depth interviews and the focus groups were able to self-identify in terms of their racial/ethnic background. A total of twenty-nine participants self-reported their ethnicity as Black or African American. Twenty-six of the participants identified as Puerto Rican. In addition, one man identified as Dominican, one woman identified as Hispanic, and another woman identified as Latina. There were also three whites and one Native American in the study sample.

Finding Hidden Risk

Project field notes and transcripts were carefully reviewed by the field coordinator, Julie Eiserman, to identify the key findings of the RARE Hartford project. Findings were defined as dominant patterns repeated through two or more sections of the data or new knowledge on HIV risk that had not been learned through prior research in Hartford. The key findings are described below.

Late-Night Culture vs. Day Culture

The project found that individuals who are out on the street, late at night, are more at risk (i.e., engage in more risky behavior) than those who are out during the day because more drug selling, drug using, hustling, and prostitution occur during this time. Moreover, given that it is dark, the lack of visibility allows illicit behavior to be more frequent, including physical and sexual violence.

Some participants reported that they had been victims of violence, especially female sex workers, who said that they occasionally get beat up or raped by their "johns" (customers) at night. The female sex workers that were interviewed stated that they often do not have a safe place to go to get off the streets temporarily, so sometimes they continue to "trick" (pick up customers for sex), when they would rather go home. Some of these women were homeless, while others simply "perform their work" too far from home to be able to go there and then walk back to the street to continue working, within a short period of time. Some of these women also mentioned that they did not have access to bathrooms and showers at night, so that they are unable to use the toilet indoors or clean themselves up. For example, a woman who has engaged in commercial sex work stated during a project focus group:

> Well, it happened to me, where a man pick[s you] up and then he doesn't want to pay you and he just throws you out of the car. Yeah, he beat me up. He broke my nose. He hit me. . . . And it was like 1 o'clock in the morning, and we do what we do, and then after he says, "You gotta get out of my car," and I say, "Why? You didn't pay me. You gotta give me my money." And he says, "I'm not gonna give you nothin'. Here's your money!" Bang!! He hit me right here. Then after that, he took all my clothes, and let me go with no clothes, with just some panties. . . .

High Level of HIV Risk at Night

It was evident from participants' accounts and answers to the interview questions that risky sexual behavior appears to occur more at night than during the day, especially because more commercial sex work occurs at this time. In addition, many of the "late-night" participants that were interviewed reported that they view themselves as being at high risk for HIV transmission. During the interviews, participants were asked, "On a scale of 1 to 10, with 10 being the most and 1 being the least, how at risk do you think you are for contracting HIV?" Most of the drug users and sex workers reported that they are 6 or higher on this scale. Participants expressed a strong concern about younger sex workers and drug users, those in their teens and early twenties, because, they said that they appear to have less knowledge about HIV and less fear of it. These participants believed that younger individuals are less likely to use condoms or be tested for HIV. Drug sellers appear to play a key role in late-night risk. Not only are these individuals peddling drugs in late-night sites, many also are engaging in sex-for-drugs exchanges with women on the street. As participants in one of the drug seller focus groups stated:

> Facilitator: What do you give that person for doing the oral sex?
> Participant 4: Whatever I can. If she'll take a nickel [bag], that's what I'll give her.
> Participant 2: As little as possible. That's why they call it tricking.
> Participant 4: Definitely no cash, you know. Strictly drugs if anything. . . .
> Participant 6: You can do better with a dime [bag] of 'caine than you can with an eight-ball 'cause if you got an eight-ball they get too greedy. If it's a dime, it's straight forward, slam, bam, thank you ma'am.
> Participant 4: And you know she ain't thinking about no AIDS. She probably go to every block and do this.

Co-Occurring Risk Behaviors

Most of the individuals that were interviewed did not fall into just one of the pre-determined risk categories, but rather into two or more categories. For example, many of the participants were drug users and sex workers; drug users and sex workers and MSM; sex workers and customers of other sex workers (these participants were mostly male); or drug users with multiple sex partners and/or were customers of sex workers. Thus, all of the sex workers that were interviewed reported that they perform sex work in exchange for crack or heroin or for money to buy these drugs. A few of them said that they also sell drugs to get money.

While most sex workers reported that they use condoms themselves, they said that they know plenty of sex workers who do not use them. Nevertheless, they mentioned a number of situations in which they consider having commercial sex without a condom. These situations include: when the customer pays more; when the customer is one of their "regulars"; when the customer "looks clean," when the customer is a professional (i.e. wearing a suit and tie); and, notably, when they are simply desperate for money, and therefore, willing to do whatever the client wants. For example, as the following excerpt from the focus group with female sex workers suggests, condom avoidance may be most frequent in commercial sex when client demand coincides with sex work need.

> Participant 2: And a lot of guys, as soon as you tell them [to use] condoms. . . .
> Participant 1: They want to pay you extra money to do it [without]. So it's hard.
> Facilitator: So what percentage of the time would you say that you're with a man and he refuses to wear one?
> Participant 1: 91%. . . .
> Participant 3: If he says "no," you already know something's going on. A lot of them say, "Well, if I want[ed] it like that (with a condom), I wouldn't be out here. They automatically assume that when they go out with a [sex worker], that she's gonna go without it, if he wants. If I want money, I'm gonna go whatever way he wants it!

In terms of sexual identity, half of the male sex workers identified as heterosexual and reported having sex with men only for money. The other half of the male sex workers identified as bisexual. The male sex workers reported having both male and female clients, while only one female sex worker reported having both female and male clients. In addition, participants reinforced findings from other studies about the frequency of exchanges of sex for drugs or money and that these exchanges occur within a wide variety of contexts and involve an array of partner dynamics. Moreover, while researchers or prevention educators might view all such exchanges as sex work or prostitution, this perception is not always shared by participants as demonstrated by this quote from the focus group with Latino MSM:

> Participant 4: There is a situation of control, that is, the [man] that has the money and the drugs is the person that decides whether [they are going to use protection] or not, and . . . [mostly], they don't want to use protection.
> Participant 3: And we are talking about . . .eighteen year old boys that are just starting to go out [to meet men]. . . . And those [men] look for those people because they are young and more vulnerable. . . .
> Participant 5: They buy things for them and influence them with drugs.

Overall, the MSM participants in the study reported that popular night locations in Hartford include gay bars/dance clubs, parks, and an adult bookstore. They reported that there are limited locations in the area for MSM to socialize together at night, and that those that exist encourage casual sex. They also said that alcohol and drugs, especially marijuana, cocaine, and ecstasy, are prevalent in the late night Gay community. The participants that we interviewed, as well as some of the providers that we interviewed who have MSM clients, reported that MSM commonly have multiple sex partners, and that some also have female partners. Some participants also stated that some MSM give money or drugs to other men in exchange for sex. They said this was especially true of some older men who want to have sex with younger men. The participants reported that many MSM still do not use condoms regularly, despite having information about the transmission of HIV. They reported that "getting drunk" at the bar plays a large role in men initiating sex, and not using a condom. The MSM participants and some providers also said that there is a lack of condoms and HIV/STI information in places that are popular among MSM, e.g. the adult bookstore. Finally, they reported that there are limited services in the area that specifically target non-gay-identified MSM; Latino, gay or bisexual-identified men; and gay, lesbian, bisexual, and transgender (GLBT) youth, especially GLBT youth who are also ethnic minorities.

Discussing condom use among MSM, a participant in the Latino MSM focus group stated:

> Some of my friends have their own partners, and they think that it is something steady and forever, so they don't see the need to use condoms. There are others that have in their mind that something can happen . . . that they may sleep with others . . . so they always use condoms.
>
> Another focus group participant stated:
>
> "I have had contact with different men. . . . And if I am not alert. . . I mean I say, "No. We have to use a condom!", and they [still] don't use them, and there's a lot of people like that. There are many people that I know that are highly educated, but also when they have their minds hot, they don't think straight, and they forget the condoms. They forget everything!

As these comments suggest, risk patterns vary in complex ways, suggesting the need for targeted intervention.

Crack Cocaine Users at Very High Risk

In particular, crack cocaine users in the study were at high risk for HIV transmission. First of all, more than half of the crack users that were interviewed also injected heroin. In addition, most of them were also sex workers. Moreover, given the short "high" associated with crack use, users report that they often spend hundreds of dollars a day to get high. Accordingly, users may have to turn many "tricks" (i.e., have sex with many customers) in one night to support their habit. Many of the male crack users and one female crack user also reported that they have both male and female customers. As one field team participant recorded in her field notes after an interview with a participant:

> He told me that people who are using drugs, particularly crack cocaine, become so consumed with their drug habit that they just don't care anymore. He says that half of them probably suspect that they are infected,

> but won't take the time to get tested. The general mindset around this behavior is that, "I don't want to know."

Finally, crack users reported that they have serious difficulty accessing inpatient treatment while they remain active users. Inquiry with local treatment providers yielded the following information: public insurance requires that crack cocaine users also use heroin or alcohol as well, or be clean (abstain from drug use) for as much as thirty days in order to enter treatment. Although they are able to access out-patient treatment, many users report that if they are not removed from their environment totally for a period of time, they will not be able to stay drug-free.

HIV Testing and Status

Most interview participants reported that they had been tested for HIV at some point during their lives. Still, interviewees emphasized that fear often prevents them and their peers from getting tested regularly or returning to get results. Three out of the thirty-one individuals who completed an interview said that they were HIV-positive. All of these individuals were sex workers. Although we did not ask about HIV status in the focus groups, two out of the thirty-one individuals who completed a focus group volunteered that they were HIV-positive, during one of the groups.

Less Exposure to Prevention Information and Services

Most of the late-night individuals that we interviewed reported that they have received HIV/AIDS information at some point in their lives. Eighty percent of the sixty-seven participants who completed the survey said that they had received HIV/AIDS information before. Yet, participants were divided in their opinions about whether there is enough HIV/AIDS information and AIDS-related services out in the Hartford community. About 65% of the survey participants said that they thought there was enough HIV/AIDS information in Hartford right now, while just over 60% said that they thought there were enough HIV/AIDS services. However, street participants in the study, as well as providers that we interviewed, reported that late-night individuals tend to sleep during the day and thus have less access/exposure to information/services, including HIV education, than those who are awake and out in the community during the day.

Less Access to Harm-Reduction Materials

While most late-night participants in the study said that generally there is a sufficient amount of free condoms available during the day in Hartford, they said that free condoms are often not available to them when they need them the most, at night. Also, they reported that there is not a sufficient amount of free, sterile syringes available during the day or night in Hartford.

Absence of Late-Night Outreach

Only three participants, including those who responded to the street surveys, reported ever having seen an outreach worker out late at night in Hartford, and one of those participants stated that this sighting occurred in a bar. The experiences of the RARE fieldworkers, while performing late-night ethnography in Hartford, support the assessment that late-night HIV-prevention outreach is not readily apparent and may not exist. None of the fieldworkers ever saw an outreach worker while they were out in the field over an eight-week period. Participants in a project focus group noted:

> Participant 1: They gotta bring it to the street corner because a lot of my peoples that's out there, that's with me, people I serve, man, they don't leave that corner for nothin' . . . If the program comes to them, maybe something could happen. . . . And the thing about it is, they can't do it during the day time because I don't make no money during the day. . . .
> Participant 3: The bottom line, more outreach period, in the hours where shit is really happening, which is realistically from 7 p.m. in the evening all the way through to the early next morning.

Recommendations

Based on the findings reported above, the field team, field coordinator, and field investigator, Merrill Singer, developed a set of recommendations for programmatic and policy changes, which were submitted to the CAWG and have become the basis, since the completion of the data collection phase of the project, of information-sharing and advocacy efforts of RARE Hartford staff. The recommendations developed in RARE Hartford were as follows:

- Creation of an all-night safe, drop-in center for women only (to minimize gender-related conflicts within center). Over the long term, we recommend the creation of a second center for men. The drop-in center should have the following four components: a) night site for distribution of condoms and other harm-reduction materials, and rapid HIV testing; b) case management and referral to drug treatment, mental health services, and other health services; c) temporary shelter for women to rest and take a shower; and d) temporary haven for sex workers and other women to escape risky/violent situations and receive crisis intervention;

- Development of new HIV-prevention programs focused on late-night, "hot spot" outreach-prevention efforts, including condom dispersal. The programs should include both field workers on the street and a mobile van which travels throughout Hartford;
- Convening of a meeting of drug treatment and AIDS-prevention providers to formulate a city-wide "bridge to treatment" plan for linking late night crack users with drug treatment and for helping them stay in treatment;
- Development of a trial late-night syringe exchange to augment the community syringe change operated during the day in Hartford;
- Formation of a prevention program that targets MSM who do not identify as gay or bisexual.

Having an Impact

One of the most significant challenges of any RARE project is having a real impact on the local setting in terms of AIDS risk and prevention/intervention efforts. It has been evident in the Hartford project that to have a meaningful effect, RARE projects cannot end with the reporting of findings to the local community advisory group. Instead, it is at this point that systematic publicity and advocacy efforts must begin, which is made especially difficult because federal funding for the RARE projects ends shortly after the final report to the advisory group occurs. Consequently, to have a real impact it is necessary to have a plan in place and the organization structure needed to support work after the formal project has ended.

This approach was possible in Hartford because the project was implemented through a community-based organization with a long track record of AIDS prevention and an infrastructure that could be used to sustain post-project efforts to translate RARE findings into meaningful changes in the city. In Hartford, beginning with the presentation of the final report to the CAWG, we have placed a strong emphasis on statewide dissemination of findings to AIDS-concerned groups, institutions, and individuals. Formal presentations have been done at the Greater Hartford Ryan White Title 1 Planning Group, which is responsible for the distribution of Ryan White Title 1 AIDS care funding in the city; the Connecticut HIV Prevention Planning Group, which sets priorities for CDC-funded AIDS prevention/intervention initiatives in the state; a number of AIDS service organizations and community organizations; several key state legislators involved in developing the state budget; and researchers and community providers at the annual science meeting of an AIDS research center. Subsequent to these meetings, the final bound project report was distributed to participants in these meetings and other concerned officials and individuals around the city and state.

Thus far, a number of promising changes have occurred as a result of the RARE Hartford Project. After two consecutive years of significant cuts in the state syringe exchange program budget, the governor of Connecticut has restored over $100,000 to the next budget for use in syringe exchange (1/3 for Hartford). Notably, RARE findings were part of the materials used to make the case for this restoration. One of the legislators who has pushed for restoring cut funds to syringe exchange program in the state has cited the need for late-night syringe exchange in a public speech to AIDS advocates following his meeting with the RARE field coordinator. The Hispanic Health Council has continued efforts to disseminate RARE findings and to advocate for the recommendations made by the project.

Thus, the Hispanic Health Council has held two meetings with the Hartford Department of Health and Human Services to develop a late-night drop-in center for women, which will include a mobile outreach team, and possibly a fixed-site needle exchange program. Discussion of this project at various community meetings has generated a lot of local "buzz" about the need for such a center. The Hispanic Health Council is continuing efforts to secure funding to realize this critical recommendation. Additionally, the Hispanic Health Council has begun discussion intended to develop a grant for HIV prevention among MSM who do not self-identify as gay/bi-sexual. Furthermore, the Hispanic Health Council is working with A Better Way Foundation (a prison and substance abuse policy reform non-profit organization) and the Alliance (a state-wide prison and substance abuse policy reform coalition) to organize a round-table discussion of key community officials from drug treatment agencies, the Department of Social Services, and the Department of Mental Health and Addiction Services to discuss barriers to in-patient treatment for active crack cocaine users.

Discussion

A primary challenge that RARE Hartford faced was the retention and availability of field team staff. Given that RARE Hartford was a late-night project with temporary, part-time staff, this was not wholly unexpected. In fact, knowing this had been a problem at some other RARE sites, we prepared for this problem by developing a pool of potential field team members. Nonetheless, during the first month of the project, we lost four members of the field team. Fortunately, we were able to quickly add two new staff members to fill some of these positions. Towards the end of the project, we lost two additional staff people. Staff left the project for several reasons, including obtaining another job with conflicting hours and concern about one's health or safety during late-night fieldwork in high-risk locations. Other staff members were asked to leave because they were not meeting the requirements of the job. Additionally, the project suffered some because field team members were not always able to follow through on their late night data collection responsibilities due to personal obligations and issues, as well as weather conditions, e.g., rain. When this occurred, we attempted to increase the hours of other staff, and/or increase the number of hours spent in the field, to insure that we were staying on schedule. In addition, because most staff members had little, if any prior training in research or note taking in the field, they required additional support from the field coordinator, expanding the demands on this position and hindering project functioning to some degree.

Overall, the project took considerably more coordination time and energy than was actually covered by available project funding. Again, because of our awareness of this issue through our familiarity with the experience of earlier RARE projects, we were able to meet this challenge through teamwork, working additional hours, and relying on the existing structure for research coordination within the Hispanic Health Council.

In terms of challenges in meeting our data collection goals, the only population for which we were unable to meet our target goal was community service providers. This was partly due to the fact that this population was recruited toward the end of the project. At that time, there were only two field staff members, other than the coordinator, who were still employed on the project. The field staff also had exhausted most of their professional contacts and staff at local agencies for completion of the surveys and interviews, before they began to recruit for the focus group. Also, providers who had completed the surveys and interviews were excluded from participating in a focus group. Recruitment for the focus group was done through an e-mail to local community providers. The team only received two positive responses to this e-mail, which was an insufficient number for a focus group. Unfortunately, at this point, the target end date for data collection was also past and the final CAWG meeting was just days away. As a result, the remaining field team members decided to stop trying to recruit providers for a focus group. The project team was able to meet all of its other data collection goals prior to the final CAWG meeting.

Finally, as data collection was being completed, it became clear that a considerable amount of work would need to be accomplished after RARE funding had ended to both disseminate project findings to AIDS policy makers, service providers, and the public and to advocate and plan for the implementation of the project's recommendations. Meeting these twin challenges has been possible because they fit with the research dissemination, public health education, program development, and community advocacy missions of the Hispanic Health Council, and thus could be folded into the daily work of our organization. Without having such a structure in place, however, it would have been difficult to aggressively support the achievement of the RARE recommendations.

Conclusion

As we move closer to the end of the third decade of the AIDS epidemic, it is important to assess the role of social and behavioral qualitative methods in AIDS research, including the utility of rapid assessment models like the RARE initiative. As participant-observers of RARE in Hartford, we have seen the value of: 1) involving service providers, activists, and policy makers in prevention studies, from the very beginning, to identify the areas of need and participate in project planning, can significantly enhance the ability of researchers to subsequently disseminate their findings broadly to appropriate audiences; 2) using a rapid assessment approach that shortens the temporal distance from the initiation of research to the reporting of findings helps to generate considerable momentum that can be used to help drive the dissemination of project findings to the community; 3) organizing research to produce specific achievable recommendations for change helps to insure that significant findings do not languish in a journal article that is never seen by programmatic staff and policy makers; 4) uniting community-based research with an advocacy orientation helps to insure that applied research be used as a tool for achieving community needs; and 5) use of qualitative methods—that produce poignant insider accounts of personal experience and behavior—increases the accessibility of findings for the community. For all of these reasons RARE Hartford Project has been a visible and increasingly impactful initiative.

References

Annie E. Casey Foundation (2003) *The Right Start for America's Newborns: A Decade of City and State Trends (1990–2000)*. Baltimore: Annie E. Casey Foundation.

Connecticut Department of Public Health (2002) *Epidemiologic Profile of HIV and AIDS*. Hartford: Connecticut Department of Public Health.

Connecticut Department of Public Health, Infectious Disease Division (2003). *Epidemiologic Profile of HIV and AIDS in Connecticut–2003*. Hartford: Connecticut Department of Public Health.

Hartford Courant, "STDs" (2001). *Hartford Courant*, April 2: 1.

Needle, R., Trotter, R.T., II, Singer, M., et al. (2003) "Rapid Assessment of the HIV/AIDS Crisis in Racial and Ethnic Minority Communities: An Approach for Timely Community Interventions." *American Journal of Public Health* 93 (6): 970–979.

Singer, Merrill (2000) "Evaluating a National AIDS Study." *Society for Applied Anthropology Newsletter* 11 (3): 3–5.

Smedley, B., Adrienne, S., Nelson A. (2003) *Unequal Treatment: Confronting Racial and Ethnic Disparities in Healthcare.* Washington: The National Academic Press.

Trinity College (2001) *A Hartford Primer and Field Guide.* Hartford, CT: Cities Data Center, Trinity College.

Trotter, R., II, Needle, R.H., Goosby, E., et al. (2001) "A Methodological Model for Rapid Assessment, Response, and Evaluation: The RARE Program in Public Health." *Field Methods* 13 (2): 137–159.

Chapter 13

RARE Research in Preventing HIV among Men Who Have Sex with Men in Pima County, Arizona

Halley Eisner-Freitas and Floyd Meeks

Scope of HIV/AIDS in Pima County, Arizona

Over the course of the AIDS epidemic in the United States, it has been well documented that men who have sex with men (MSM) have higher mortality rates from HIV/AIDS than all other groups combined. In Pima County, AZ, MSM are assumed to be less than 5% of the total population yet make up more than 60% of those infected with HIV/AIDS (ADHS Office of HIV/AIDS Epidemiological Record, 2003). For the total number of HIV/AIDS cases reported in Pima County from 1998 to 2002, 63% were self-identified as MSM (57% - MSM, 6% MSM/IDU). The actual MSM rates could even be higher as 84% of all HIV/AIDS cases in Pima County are males and some men who self-identified simply as heterosexual (6%) or IDUs (22%) may also have been involved with MSM.

In other regions in the United States, AIDS has disproportionately affected populations of color. Racial and ethnic populations account for 25% of the total U.S. population, but represent more than 50% of the cumulative U.S. AIDS cases. Of the newly reported AIDS cases in 1998, more than 65% were among African American (46%) and Hispanic (20%) adults (Needle et al. 2003). In Pima County, African Americans have also been disproportionately affected as they make up only 3% of the total population in Pima County, but are 13% of the total HIV/AIDS cases. Figure 1 illustrates that HIV/AIDS rates among all ethnicities except African Americans in Pima County are fairly consistent with their demographic profiles.

Figure 13.1: HIV/AIDS in Pima County by Ethnicity, ADHS 2003

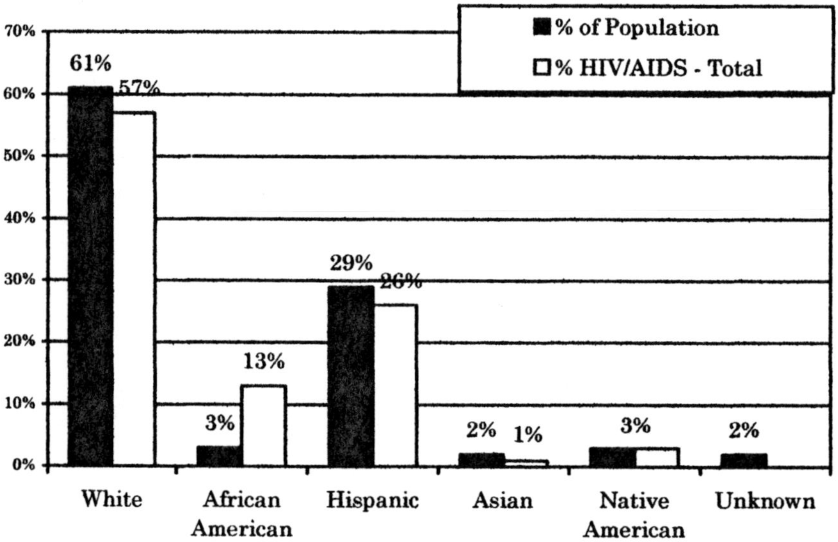

Source: Pima County Health Department.

Among MSM, the epidemiological record reveals that except for African Americans, the overall HIV/AIDS rates are also proportionally represented by ethnicity. Figure 2 shows the breakdown of MSM by ethnicity in Pima County from 1998 to 2002 for both HIV and AIDS. African American MSM show the greatest disparity of new HIV infection in relation to their population in Pima County (ADHS, Office of HIV/AIDS, Epidemiological Record, 2003). Additionally, Latino MSMs show a higher rate of AIDS infection in relation to new HIV infections. Pima County Health Department testing and counseling employees contend that it is common for Latino MSM not to get tested for HIV until they show signs of illness (personal communication). This is because of various factors including lack of health care insurance, low priority for preventive health care activities, concerns about legal or immigration status and a fear of an HIV-positive test.

Figure 13.2: HIV/AIDS in Pima County among MSM by Ethnicity

N = 446, 1998–2002, ADHS 2003

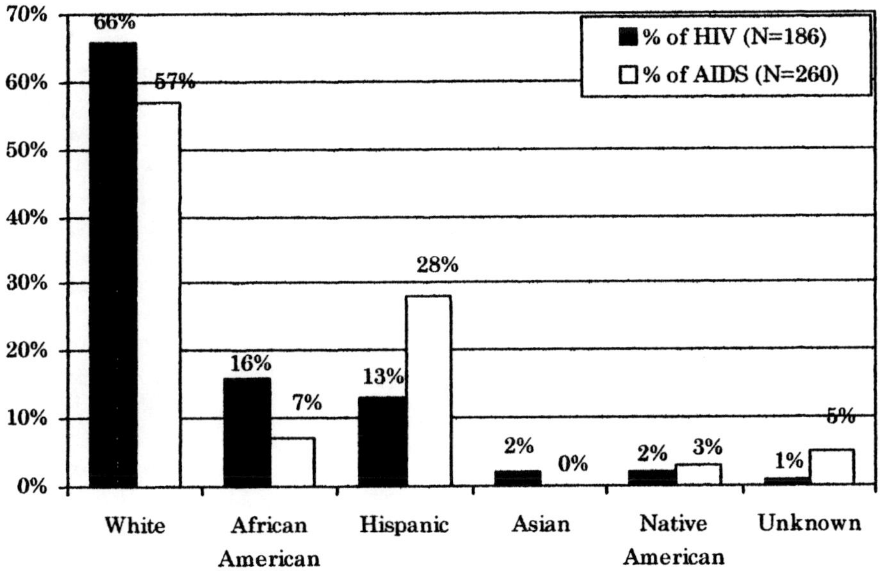

Source: Pima County Health Department.

The epidemiological record also shows that men over the age of 30 in Pima County have the highest rates of new HIV infections over the last five years (ADHS Office of HIV/AIDS, 2003). Furthermore, MSM between thirty-one and forty years of age make up 42% of the newly diagnosed HIV/AIDS cases.

In Pima County, AZ, MSM continue to be at greatest risk for getting infected with HIV. Moreover, within this MSM subgroup, men of color and/or men over thirty years old are getting infected at a higher rate than other subgroups. Based on these findings, the Tucson RARE Project has targeted MSM over thirty with an emphasis on men of color.

AIDS among Gay Men in Pima County, AZ.

In the 1970s, gay men in medium and larger cities throughout the U.S. were socialized in an environment where multiple sexual partners represented an affirmation of gay identity. With the impact of AIDS and fear that sexual pleasure symbolized death during the late 1980s, a new paradigm of sexual monogamy emerged as a strategy to be sexual without getting infected. This ideology of selective or reduced sexual activity posed tremendous conflict to gay culture in Pima County, Arizona, because a primary value in local gay culture was sexual pursuit with diverse partners. During this time, risk for AIDS in the gay community had been equated with 'promiscuity' and those men who previously had been considered 'liberated' by enjoying multiple sexual partners were now judged as 'irresponsible' or 'unhealthy.' By the 1990s, gay culture had successfully resisted these heterosexist moralities by re-sanctioning multiple partners as a norm in social networks. Local AIDS service organizations responded by promoting a sex-positive approach of negotiated safety through condom use (Freitas 1995). In the early 2000s, the development of new pharmaceutical technologies changed the AIDS disease landscape from an acute to a chronic disease. Antiviral therapies dramatically changed the way MSM thought about living with HIV/AIDS in Tucson. AIDS was no longer perceived as an imminent death threat, but rather as a disease similar to other life-long chronic conditions such as diabetes (Freitas 1997).

Although the advent of antiviral therapies changed how gay men perceive HIV/AIDS in Pima County, basic prevention messages for MSM have not been altered. Among local AIDS service organizations, the prevention message most consistently promoted for this population has been to use condoms to avoid contact with HIV (Southern Arizona AIDS Foundation, personal communication 2003). However, condom use traditionally has not been perceived as desirable by the majority of gay men involved in ethnographic research in Pima County over the last ten years, despite various AIDS service organizations' attempts to make them 'sexy'. Condoms have been used in situations (only when they were perceived to be necessary) by many gay men who were well-educated about the risks of HIV/AIDS and 'knew better' (Freitas 1996, 1997). Recent reports from the Center for Disease Control have revealed that between 1999–2001, new HIV diagnoses among MSM have increased 14% in the U.S. due in part to the availability of new antiviral therapies (Gross 2003).

HIV Risk among MSM: Public Sex Environments

Before the devastation of AIDS, public sex was perceived as a 'gesture of communion' (Clatts 1999) and resistance to mainstream culture among gay men. But as unrestricted sex became recognized as the primary vehicle for the spread of AIDS, public sex became stigmatized as high-risk sex. As Clatts observed (1999), unregulated sex has been medicalized as sexual addiction, identified with a personality type that is clinically termed 'compulsive and out of control' and as maladjusted. Similar diagnostic images attend the contexts in which some men find male sexual partners—bars, bathhouses, bookstores, public parks and bathroom "tearooms." These are places represented as conducive to "impersonal sex," a term that in itself is loaded with cultural meanings denoting something "strange," "deviant" and "dangerous." Public sex environments historically have been equated with deviancy and are therefore perceived to attract high-risk individuals including non-gay identified MSMs, sex addicts or gay/bisexual men who feel that they cannot attract other MSM in other gay-centric settings.

Humphreys's landmark study on tearoom sex (1970) set the standard of knowledge of who used public restrooms for sex. His research revealed that 38% of his subjects were married, 24% were bisexual (and married), 24% were covert homosexuals and 14% were openly gay. The common thread among all of these men was that they wanted some form of orgasm-producing action that was less lonely than masturbation and less involving than a love relationship (Sieber 2003). The tearooms contained a distinct culture with a code of verbal silence so that body language and hand signals were the primary means of communication. Recent research among public sex environments (PSE) (Brown 2003), cast doubt upon the assumption pioneered by Humphreys that public sex is always an anonymous and impersonal event. Instead, Brown's research suggests that these environments serve as a place for MSM to congregate with others like themselves and form a sense of community with one another. Leap (1999) concurs that PSEs can create a communication network for MSM who do not identify with public gay culture and/or for gay men as an additional resource for sexual contact.

Binson et al. (2001) discovered that about half the MSM in their sample (N=2,478) reported going to a sex venue such as a bathhouse or public cruising areas. Multi-venue users and bath house patrons were more likely than cruisers to be HIV-positive, to have had a STD, to report using poppers, ecstasy, methamphetamines and other party drugs and to engage in unprotected anal sex. In other words, HIV-positive men remain sexually active, seek sexual partners in the same settings as uninfected men and are more likely to engage in unprotected anal intercourse in a public setting. Additionally, the more venues an individual uses for sex, the higher the likelihood that he will engage in unprotected sex.

Theoretical Considerations for the Tucson RARE Project

This research uses an innovative method to examine HIV risk in MSM by shifting the focus from risky people to risky places. The environment becomes the primary locus of intervention rather than trying to change or label individual behavior. By identifying the place-based networks, interventions such as condom distribution or outreach could be developed that reach the targeted population just before they actually have sex (Weir et al. 2003).

The three most popular approaches in the study of human illness found in social and cultural settings in anthropology are (Hahn 1999, in Maners, 1999b):

- An ecological/evolutionary approach focuses on human adaptation to the environment as the main determinant of illness and health.
- A cultural theory approach which emphasizes beliefs, values and customs as the primary determinants of sickness and health.
- A political/economic approach contends that economics and other relations of power are the main determining factors in sickness and health.

Thorough ethnographic analyses can use all approaches in contextualizing health problems and linking individual or micro decision-making to larger macro social forces. Traditionally, however, one theory usually emerges as the most applicable perspective to frame an analysis. Because this research is focused upon the interplay between the environment and risk-taking behaviors, the ecological approach was emphasized. However, the cultural theory approach was important to describe the changing perceptions of what it means to be HIV-positive in the gay community and to a lesser degree the political/economic approach was important to examine the effects of homophobia and oppression among the gay community in this analysis.

Methods

Five methods were used in this research: 1) gatekeeper surveys, 2) observation and mapping, 3) street intercept surveys, 4) focus groups, and 5) cultural expert interviews (focus groups and interviews were not reported here).

Gatekeeper Surveys

The purpose of the Brief Gatekeeper Survey (BGS) was to guide the development of the RARE research questions. The BGS was conducted and analyzed prior to the two 24-hour observations or the question development on the Cultural Expert Interview and the Focus Groups. The survey was administered to twelve men and eight women who worked in Native and African American and/or gay communities, health care including HIV-prevention staff and outreach workers, as well as city staff officials and HIV-positive persons. The questions were:

- Who do you think is at greatest risk for HIV in Tucson?
- What is it about their behavior that puts them at risk?
- Where do you think men in Tucson meet other men for sex?

Observation and Mapping

Two 24-hour continuous observations were conducted during the first month of the research. The locations selected were chosen because of their consistent use by MSM and were:

- Greasewood Park: a public sex environment (PSE) in a desert park containing miles of dirt hiking trails; 4th Avenue: a six-city block corridor in downtown Tucson where a collection of businesses caters to the gay community.

Street Intercept Surveys

The Street Intercept Survey (SIS) was developed to gather data from a large sample size of MSM about locations and perceived risk for HIV. The survey was designed as a short, anonymous survey lasting about 10 minutes. A total of two hundred SIS's were collected at various gay bars, bookstores, parks, health-related organizations, coffee shops and private parties. The four basic questions that were asked on the SIS are the following:

- Can you describe for me the different locations where men find other male sexual partners? Please list all the places you know of where men meet each other for sex?
- Which places are the three most popular for men looking for sex with men? Why?
- Of the places you listed, where do you actually hook up with men? Why?
- Where would you feel most at risk for getting infected with HIV?

Summary of Findings

Findings from the three most popular places of HIV risks are reported here. New locations are explored; they become increasingly well known and then become identified as gay-sex areas by non-gays and then decline in favor of new, less-known locations.

Greasewood Park

> I had a schedule that I could follow because I was a regular. Until you become a regular you don't really know when the best time is to go. A lot of

> it is opportunity and that's part of the thrill of cruising. You never know [who you will meet] whereas in a bar, it's pretty predictable.

Greasewood Park is a desert oasis surrounded by new housing developments in the foothills of west Tucson. Dirt trails for hiking or jogging crisscross the low hills and arroyos. Despite its convenient location to downtown and large size, the park appears to be infrequently used by non-MSM patrons. During the RARE observation for example, about 10% of park patrons were considered to be non-MSM. The Greasewood Park observation began on a Wednesday morning at 5:00 a.m. and ended on Thursday morning at 5:00 a.m. MSM activity was presumed to be lower during the weekdays than during the weekends.

Observation was focused primarily on the MSM who frequented the park. MSM park patrons did attempt to make contact with team members by following them around, but field team members tried not to interact much with them other than to signal that they were not interested in sex. One field team member was solicited by a naked man bent over a park table and who held up condoms in his hand. He asked the field team member, "do you want to fuck me? I have condoms."

Communication patterns among the MSM park patrons observed by the field team were largely non-verbal and relied heavily on eye contact and upon following one another. This 'culture of silence' has been well documented in the literature (Humphreys 1970). The majority of men arrived at the park alone and left alone, inferring that most of their sexual contact occurred at the park. Hundreds of used condoms and lube packets were found discarded in the desert or in the trash cans near the parking lot. It was unclear however how long the condoms had been out there as some were already decomposed. Anal sex appeared to be a common activity in this environment based on direct observations of the field team members as well as evidence of discarded condoms that were still wet along the trails. Other research in public sex environments argues that anonymity among MSM is not a dominant feature. Rather, a loose social network exists in that they know each other on some level and have some form of ongoing social interaction (Clatts 1999). Field team members observed on a couple of occasions that some men appeared to recognize each other and hooked up quickly with one another.

Along 4th Avenue

> At the bars, you have the opportunity to talk and to explore more and find out more about your partner to assess your risk. [If you are in] a Macy's bathroom or a public sex environment at noon, people want to, you know, fuck and get fucked, get blown and blow.

Fourth Avenue is a commercial district that caters to non-mainstream consumers. Located half way between downtown and the University of Arizona, 4th

Avenue offers local restaurants, bars and coffee shops and independent retail stores. The most popular gay bar, 'It's About Time' or IBT is on 4th Avenue as well as a gay-centric coffee shop next door, the Rainbow Planet. Both of these businesses were located in the four blocks designated for observation. A gay youth drop-in center called the Lounge, and Wingspan, a GLBT community center are also located within a block of IBT. IBT has been at this location for twelve years and serves as a focal point that has attracted other gay-centric businesses and organizations.

The observation along 4th Avenue began on a Friday afternoon at 5:00p.m. and ended on Saturday afternoon at 5:00p.m. By evening, groups were congregated in the restaurants and coffee shops made up of both gay and non-gay patrons. By 11:00 p.m., IBT was doing a brisk business. Small groups of underage gay/bisexual youth were observed in the gay coffee shop next door or milling up and down the street. Illegal activity such as selling drugs or sex work was not observed. Additionally, no sex among MSM was observed inside the bar, in the streets or alleys of the observational zone.

Other Locations

> Sex parties are when you meet on the Internet. My ex-boyfriend used to invite all kind of guys over, up to 10–15 guys in the house, all having sex, never protected sex. Everybody knew that nobody had a condom on. So many people were fucked up on drugs that they knew they couldn't come. You couldn't come because you were on crystal meth and so you had a false sense of security that someone that was fucking you couldn't come and it would take forever. So when they pulled out, you're like 'okay, well he didn't come in me so I must be okay'.

The first question on the survey asked about different locations for sex and was designed to be an ice-breaker to help men think about MSM sexual locations. Respondents were to list as many locations that they knew of off the top of their heads. More than sixty-five locations were listed in the Tucson area where MSM go to find sex in addition to eleven more locations in nearby cities including Nogales and Phoenix. Three cities in Sonora, Mexico and two in Southern California were also listed. The average number of locations described by each respondent was ten. The reason for the high number of responses is that most respondents listed multiple bars, bookstores, parks or Internet sites. IBT's bar was the most commonly chosen venue of all with 78% of respondents listing it as a place where men find sexual partners. The most common venues that more than half of respondents recalled were: IBT's (78%), Greasewood Park (67%), Gay.com (64%), Venture-N (53%) and Caesar's Bookstore (51%).

The Three Most Popular Places

> People go to bathhouses because they're so horny and normally, it involves alcohol or drugs, especially later at night. Whereas if you're on the Internet or you're at a bar, you have more of an opportunity to think about what you're doing and look at the person more closely. It's not so impersonal.

Although a large selection of locations exists where MSM go to find sex, some are perceived to be more popular than others. When asked, "which places are the three most popular for men looking for sex with men," the three most commonly cited places for all gay-identified men over twenty-one years of age, regardless of ethnicity or age in order of popularity were: bars (81%), internet (53%), and parks (48%).

Bars were perceived to be the most popular, with 81% respondents, because they represented a 'gay friendly' environment where men can socialize with other gay men. According to respondents, the atmosphere was communal and represented a central gathering place for gay men to be themselves and feel safe. Other reasons why bars were perceived to be popular were that they attracted lots of gay men, and alcohol and drugs were readily available.

The Internet was also popular with 53% of respondents because of the continuous availability in finding sexual partners. According to respondents, the venue was set up so that men can interact easily and quickly. They preferred the Internet because they could find sexual partners from the privacy of their home and then meet their partners for sex in discreet locations. Respondents also liked the profiles accessible on the Internet so that they could match their sexual interests with others.

Parks were perceived to be popular by 48% of respondents because of the easy and immediate access to sex. The anonymity and non-verbal communication was desired according to respondents and it was tacitly understood that the only reason to hook up was for sex. Parks offered multiple and diverse partners constantly. Additionally, some parks were large enough to offer enough privacy so that MSM could engage in all types of sexual activities, including anal sex.

Bisexual men were slightly different in their responses than gay men in that they felt the three most popular places to hook up with MSM were in bars primarily, followed by parks and bookstores. Bookstores were popular for this subpopulation because they were open 24 hours, provided an easy access to lots of other MSM who want sex and some bookstores had gay friendly clerks who would help them hook up or warn them if trouble arises.

In summary, the places that respondents had described as risky for exposure to HIV were also popular 'gay friendly' environments where MSM socialized and hooked up with sexual partners.

Figure 13.3. Where would you feel most at risk for getting infected by HIV? Street Intercept Survey, N = 200

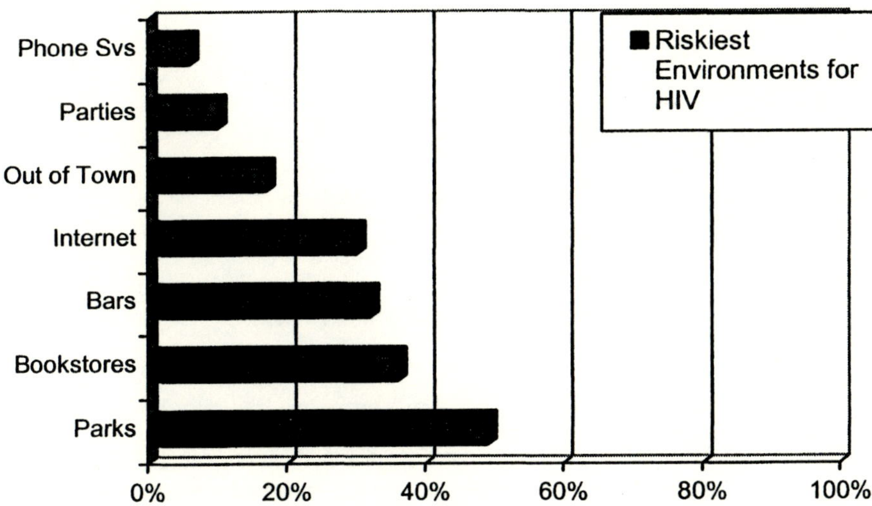

The respondents were aware that the environments that they used to hook up for sex were also risky environments. This data was matched to the smaller sample size of the cultural expert interviews (N = 27) and the focus groups (N = 39) for comparability of themes. Data from the SIS's, CEI's and focus groups about perceptions of risk for HIV in different locations where MSM hook up for sex were all very similar.

Sexual Compulsion and Addiction

> When I am in a binge situation, I just rent [porn] videos because it's too much to go out all the time. Especially when I was doing drugs and I would have twenty guys on the weekend. I can't let myself do that anymore. So, during like a five-day binge, I may actually go out twice, you know. Well, max, three or four times. It just depends.

Sexual compulsion and addiction arose as other reasons for high risk behavior among some MSM. Experts felt that a primary reason that parks were considered high risk was because of the compulsive nature of the MSM who go there. One expert explained,

> The guys who are married and identify as straight or bisexual in the parks are at highest risk because it's a sexually obsessive situation for them.

Public sex environments were defined by experts as being linked to sexual compulsion because sex can be found immediately and anonymously. MSM were not concerned about developing a reputation for being a 'pig' (someone who has frequent 'raunchy' sex with multiple partners) because they were outside of the bar culture where much of the labeling and social/sexual conformity is produced. Additionally, a stigma was attached to finding sex in parks rather than in other more mainstream settings such as gay bars. The stigma assumed that MSM seek sex out in parks as a last resort because they were unattractive, old, closeted, unsocial and/or could not find partners at the bars. The highest-risk locations were believed to be PSE's where MSM could engage in anal sex. Experts expressed that for sexually addicted men in PSE's, the sexual compulsion ultimately takes priority over condom use. One expert described the atmosphere in the Phoenix bathhouses as compulsive in an uncontrollable or animalistic way. He said,

> Bathhouses are very animalistic. It's very spontaneous and very instant. You don't think and that's the problem. I don't make excuses for it, but I let the animalistic part take over. I don't think animals really think about what they're doing, they just do it. And that is how I approach sex. It's very violent for me, fast, hard and quick.

Testing Behavior

> In the past when I was getting tested, I was having much safer sex. I grew up in the era where I thought you could get HIV from anything. I swore I would never have unsafe sex again, but here I am like seven years later and I've had unprotected sex a million times. It's because sex is such a powerful thing because when it's in the heat of the moment, you're fucked up on your drugs you don't care. You care the second after you come. You just lie there and you think I wish I could go back in time. And then you get tested less. A lot less.

Knowing one's own HIV status has long been a cornerstone of prevention. This research has confirmed previous work among MSM in Pima County that the knowledge of one's HIV status reduces the transmission of HIV (Freitas, 1996). Lack of consistent testing is often a response to the fear of being infected with HIV. For some men, it is better not to know one's status than to deal with the emotional consequences of HIV-positive test results. As one expert admitted,

> Interviewer: When was the last time you got tested?
> Expert: In 1998 or 1999.
> Interviewer: So what's kept you from getting tested again?

> Expert: Well, nothing's happened to me so far. I'm still alive and well. Based on what I've told you, I should be dead by now.

Because some men are reluctant to test regularly, they often discover their HIV status when they have been hospitalized for another illness. In Pima County, almost half of newly reported HIV/AIDS cases are men receiving their initial HIV-positive diagnosis (ADHS 2003).

Gay Life Cycle

> Older gay men who lived through the first wave of the AIDS epidemic are the people who are most at risk because they have suffered multiple losses of their friends, their core group. Many of them might have clinical depression or some unresolved grief. With me, 80% of my social circle was infected and between 1988 and 1994, we buried everybody. There wasn't time to grieve one person before another person was in the hospital and dying. It just wears on you time after time, after time. By 1994, I was so fried and so depressed I just didn't care anymore. I was overly saturated with death and dying. I had some guilt that I was not infected. Being HIV negative was a whole big ball of wax for me because all of my friends who were positive and died had fewer sex partners than I did.

A sense of fatalism emerged during these interviews related to how long gay men want to live, how and when they would get AIDS, how much they had given up socially to live 'out' in public as gay, and the fatigue of living through the succession of AIDS-related deaths in the gay community. In addition to these feelings, experts now expected to live longer than just until their thirties or forties due to improved anti-viral therapies. The impact of the more effective medications have allowed gay men to believe that they have a 'longer lease on life' and that they could once again start planning for the future. One expert explained,

> Even though more people are being affected [by HIV], it's not in the media. I mean the media may have a blurb about it, but people feel safer because they rely on technology. And I think a lot of men over thirty have a real belief that there will be a cure. Well, that's a very false sense of hope. They think a cure might be around the corner, so they can engage in riskier sex. They think the meds are really good and will help you live. So, if you're thirty you can live an extra 10–15 years, not a bad life sentence. . . . But you hate [thinking about] being in your fifties and sixties when you're thirty.

Over the course of the interviews and focus groups, a common theme emerged that could be defined as a 'life cycle' for gay men. This life cycle was a response to a combination of factors including the devastation of AIDS in the gay community, the emphasis on youth and beauty, a sense of fatalism that

AIDS is inevitable, and a renewed feeling of hope that HIV is a manageable disease as marketed by the antiviral medication advertising from pharmaceutical companies.

During a discussion on the impact of advertising on the gay community, one expert insightfully noted that the pharmaceutical companies "are not only targeting people that are already HIV-positive with the HIV meds advertising; they are targeting HIV negative individuals as well." Indeed, experts express the hope that AIDS has finally been tamed by medical science and is no longer something to dread if contracted. However, some experts, especially those who were HIV-positive, felt that the advertising was misleading and contrived. One expert complained,

> Look at those people they have advertising those drugs!! Uh huh!! And there're some cuties. And they can hang glide!! And trust me, you don't want nobody HIV-positive hang gliding over you because he'd probably shit all over you because of the meds. [Because of] one medication I [felt as if I] lived in the bathroom. It felt like my behind was on fire. It was always liquid, sometimes eight, nine times a day.

And another,

> I don't think people understand it's not as easy as taking a pill. It's just this perception [from] all of the fake advertising like the young gay guy on the hilltop. My friend, he ended up in the hospital when he took this particular cocktail. They took him off it right away. He spent two weeks out of work just because he tried taking these drugs.

The aggressive antiviral therapy medication advertising has resulted in trivializing living with AIDS. The overall perception of cultural experts was that HIV was now just another chronic disease similar to diabetes or a heart condition. One expert summarized that HIV was no longer perceived to be a 'big deal' because the gay community wants desperately to feel hopeful after 15 long years of living with death.

Recommendations

The Recommendations section is divided into four sections: the need to re-think HIV prevention/intervention, agency collaboration recommendations, RARE methodology recommendations and recommended future research. The first two sections are designed to spark innovative HIV programming in Pima County, the third section is to improve the overall RARE approach in other cities across the nation and the last section is to encourage an impetus for continued ethnographic research among high-risk populations.

The following recommendations are provided to guide HIV-prevention and intervention planning in Pima County:

Recommendation 1: There is need for multiple messages targeted to diverse populations.

This research supports recommendations provided by Huebner (2001) in Phoenix that targeting gay bars in combination with one or more other locations increases the percentage of high-risk men that can be reached. The Internet, PSE's, sex clubs and bookstores are important locations to reach out to high-risk MSM. Outreach must continue in bars but should also expand to the Internet, PSE's and bookstores and sex clubs. For example, some MSM who frequent PSE's may not self-identify as gay and therefore would need information that is not 'gay-centric' or uses 'gay' in its terminology. Additionally, some MSM in PSEs may benefit most from intervention that is largely non-verbal to fit into the sub-culture, but is also supportive and informative. Conversely, MSM who frequent bars and self-identify as gay may benefit more from normative strategies for change with gay-centric messages and face-to-face interactions.

Timing is also a critical part of being able to reach the target population. For PSE locations, certain times of day and night are busier than others. According to this research, those times are: 1) early mornings and afternoons (evening in summer time) in parks; 2) afternoons and late evenings for bookstores; 3) evenings into the early hours of the morning for internet users: and 4) evenings for the Phoenix bathhouses.

Recommendation 2: Keep the AIDS prevention message fresh and relevant.

The greatest challenge is to keep the message fresh since men have always negotiated their way through safe sex. The majority of MSM know how HIV is spread and that condoms reduce the risk for HIV. Older men in Pima County disproportionately account for new HIV infections. A behavioral change among MSMs over thirty years of age has occurred over the last few years and can be attributed to the belief that AIDS can be successfully managed with antiviral therapies and a sense of condom fatigue. The internet is a new and convenient technology to meet MSM for sex, and bathhouses and PSEs are again acceptable places to look for anal sex. Possible themes that came out of this research are the following:

- HIV is not inevitable
- Being gay does not equal having AIDS
- The meds are great but having AIDS will still compromise health and vitality
- Growing older is desirable and respectable
- Your community is your family
- Embrace diversity including age, body shape, color, etc.

- Sexual pleasure does not need to include drugs and alcohol (sober sex as a value).

New messages need to be developed based upon these themes to keep up with changed social values and sexual pursuit patterns of MSM.

Recommendation 3: Outreach must be conducted in public sex environments.

Parks are more risky because more anal sex goes on in parks than in bookstores. Bookstore booths are too small for two men to have anal sex without making enough noise to draw attention.

Public sex environments such as parks and bookstores will need one-to-one outreach that provides basic informational messages about HIV/AIDS that is not gay-specific to attract MSM who do not identify as gay.

This recommendation can be implemented by distributing health information on car windshields. This information should include other places that MSM can meet for sex as well as a list of programs, clubs, organizations and services that cater to MSM. Information should also be provided on legal and illegal sexual behavior in parks and other public places. Condoms should be distributed as well. The PCHD mobile health van should be taken to targeted parks and bookstores so that MSM could get tested for STDs and AIDS.

MSMs should be encouraged to leave the park and have sex in private. This recommendation, however, carries the consequence of losing contact with the fragile target population network. As Prieur (Chng and Geliga-Vargas) noted, "those lacking social support for their sexuality find comfort and security in anal intercourse as a means of making contact with others like them. Sex is an act deeply embedded and influenced by the social context in which it occurs. Interventions targeting sexual behaviors of non-gay identified MSM that ignore the cultural context in which these men interact are doomed to fail." However, the benefit of encouraging MSM to have sex in private locations could result in increased conversation and sexual negotiation among potential partners.

Outreach for non-gay identified MSM in parks, bookstores must be different in approach than gay-centered outreach. Messages need to de-stereotype gay in PSE outreach messages so that different types of MSM can relate to the message. These messages might also be appropriate for gay men who frequent PSE's because of their generalized feelings of ambivalence about their affiliation with the gay community.

Recommendation 4: HIV/AIDS prevention outreach is necessary on the Internet.

This venue is the newest and most rapidly growing technology to find sex with other men. Innovative strategies need to be developed to respond to this important communication resource. It is recommended that outreach workers contact other AIDS service organizations that are currently conducting outreach to learn what are the most successful strategies. Possible interventions could include pop-up ads, outreach workers cruising on-line and providing information or setting up a specific web page for Tucson with specific links, other desirable information about sexual preference and safer sex messages. For example, an alternative website to barebackcity.com could be developed locally that advocates for safer sex practices for men who want to hook up with other men. This website could use similar sensational strategies that popularized barebackcity.com in a deliberate movement to provide a place for men to hook up with other men interested in practicing safer sex.

> Recommendation 5: There is a need for specific HIV-prevention messages in gay bars.

This research has raised the premise that the closer the timing of condom distribution is to the sexual activity, the higher the likelihood that it may actually be used. It is therefore recommended that condoms or 'fuck kits' be passed out as the bars close and patrons are leaving the bar with their partners. Additionally, messages in the bar environment should not focus on HIV because the gay population is already well-versed in what AIDS is and how the disease is passed. Rather, a media campaign should explore core normative issues that emerged in the research such as the concept of a diverse gay community, the acceptability of growing older, addiction (drugs, alcohol, sex), the value of relationships, etc. These messages should be provided through multiple venues (posters, dee-jay, entertainment, outreach, etc.). There are a number of key issues that must be addressed in a social marketing campaign for gay men in bars. They are:

Compulsive Behavior and Addiction

Compulsive behavior and addiction were themes linked frequently with sexual behavior. Gay culture supports the cognitive separation between sex as a physical release and sex as an expression of emotional commitment. It is recommended that increased information, education and other intervention strategies are provided to MSM about the effects of drug and alcohol abuse and/or sexual addiction and that the link is made between drug use and increased risk to HIV because of a lack of condom use.

'Gay Community' Membership

'Gay community' membership is fluid and MSM in this research had mixed feelings about their level of commitment. Many MSM do not feel as though they fit in because they do not conform to these stereotypes of what they perceive gay to be. As a result, they have ambivalent feelings about their commitment to gay community identification. It is recommended to develop diverse messages for different types of MSM through a media campaign, small group discussions, outreach and larger forums to expand the definition of gay community.

The Concept of a Preferred Life Cycle

The concept of a preferred life cycle arose as a dominant theme throughout the interviews and focus groups. Many experts felt that an acceptable life cycle for gay men ended around sixty years of age. In this paradigm, it would not be a tragedy if a man becomes infected with HIV in his thirties. Part of this life cycle paradigm may also be influenced by the burgeoning acceptance that having HIV is no longer considered a big deal, a concept marketed heavily by the anti-viral medication pharmaceutical companies. It is recommended that a media campaign be implemented to visually deconstruct the foundations of this life cycle preference. Information gathering should be a central component to learn what imagery other AIDS programs have developed around the country. A working group should be organized to choose which images would be most applicable in this community.

MSM Have a Host of Sexual Relationships

MSM have a host of sexual relationships that should be recognized in prevention messages including monogamous relationships, open relationships and a series of short-term or anonymous sexual encounters. Messages need to address the social and sexual well-being of MSM in each of these relationship types. For example, for MSM in committed relationships, they may need skills or support in how to navigate safer sex with a partner(s). Workshops, lectures, dinner parties in individual's homes, etc., are recommended to create environments where MSM are encouraged to discuss the various negotiation skills that MSM need to maintain safe and nurturing relationships.

> Recommendation 6: Collaboration is essential between the Tucson Police Department and the GLBT Commission.

The Tucson Police Department has collaborated with the GLBT community for more than a decade and informs key organizations prior to raids in the parks. Gay men are then often informed of police presence either through the informal network or an announcement placed in the Observer, the local GLBT newspaper. Gay men therefore have specialized knowledge that MSM who do not affiliate with gay community do not have access to. Using undercover police in the parks will most likely result in arrests of MSM who are married and/or men of color who do not affiliate with the gay community. The social recriminations for these men to be caught and then possibly be registered as sex offenders are enormous and could devastate their carefully constructed and separate heterosexual and homosexual lives.

It is recommended that:

- The Pima County Health Department, in collaboration with the GLBT commission, should develop an informational brochure about public sex. This brochure can be distributed by uniformed police to individuals who appear to be loitering near known public sex environments during their routine surveillance of public parks.
- The GLBT commission should gather information on the procedure to change the legal case definition of MSM who are arrested in parks from a criminal to a civil case.
- The PCHD, Southern Arizona AIDS Foundation and the PCHD should collaborate with the Tucson Police Department to explore the feasibility of developing a diversion program for MSM who have been arrested for public sex in parks. This diversion program would be modeled after the Utah program where MSM must attend an eight week program with a therapist to avoid registering as a sex offender.
- Plain clothed police should not be used to arrest MSM in public settings because it disproportionately affects non self-identified MSM.

Recommendation 7: Increased HIV testing needs to be increasingly available for MSMs.

Knowing one's HIV status is critical in maintaining safer sex behaviors. It is recommended that increased testing is encouraged by making it more convenient and more available for MSM. It is recommended that:

- Pima County Health Department needs to start HIV/AIDS drop-in testing at different locations, in addition to the existing scheduled appointments.
- Testing in gay bars should occur during peak hours (e.g., 9 p.m.–12 p.m.).
- AIDS service outreach workers need training in rapid HIV field testing so that county workers do not have to participate (reluctantly) in late hour bar testing.
- Walk-in testing availability should be increased in gay-centric coffee shops and organizations. Testing should be held at regular intervals and at the same locations to provide consistency.
- A mobile van testing calendar should be posted in key environments such as in bars, coffee shops, park bulletin boards, bookstores, gay newspapers, etc., that describe when and where testing will occur.
- 'I got tested' stickers should be distributed to everyone who has been tested to promote a positive social norm that testing is a politically

and/or socially desirable activity similar to the stickers associated with voting, "I voted" or giving blood, "I gave blood today."

Finally, there is a need for other agency collaborations. Collaboration is critical among key social service agencies in the fight against AIDS. It is recommended that the following agencies/organizations work together to develop an interdependent plan of communication and intervention to heighten a network of inter- and intra-agency investment in reducing AIDS. The Pima County Health Department, Wingspan Community Center, Southern Arizona AIDS Foundation, GLBT commission, Tucson Police Department, TIHAN, COPE/CODAC/AA, counselors/therapists and the mayor's office are recommended to serve as core members. However, the collaboration should not be limited only to these agencies, especially if other agencies show interest. The proposed involvement and recommendations for core agencies are the following:

- Pima County Health Department could staff HIV outreach workers and a program manager who would frequent PSEs, bars and bookstores and go onto the Internet to provide HIV/AIDS information and education, support, condoms and testing opportunities. Additionally, the program manager would be responsible for maintaining regular collaboration meetings and facilitating the sharing of information and resources.
- Wingspan could broaden the definition of 'gay community' so that it is more inclusive of men and women who have same-gender sex, but may not affiliate with the stereotyped 'gay community.'
- Southern Arizona AIDS Foundation can develop the social marketing campaign for MSM to be delivered in multiple venues with diverse messages.
- GLBT commission can develop policies on legal issues for MSM in PSEs and write informational brochures on public sex that the Tucson Police Department can pass out while on duty.
- Tucson Police Department in collaboration with the GLBT commission can distribute educational materials for all people who have sex in public settings.
- TIHAN could provide spiritual guidance to MSMs.
- COPE/CODAC/AA can provide substance abuse intervention opportunities for MSMs.
- Counselors/therapists must be available to provide pro bono counseling services to MSM in crisis.
- The mayor's office can provide political support for HIV/AIDS prevention and intervention programs.

References

Binson, D., Woods, W.J., Pollack, L., et al. (2001) "Differential HIV Risk in Bathhouses and Public Cruising Areas." American Journal of Public Health, 91: 1482–1486

Bradbury M.C. (1999) Resurgence of Syphilis in Seattle Traced to Bathhouses and Sex Clubs. Seattle Gay News Online, http://sgn.org/Archives/sgn. 9.10.99/syp.htm.

Brown, M. (2003) Thanks Buddy: Gay and Bisexual Men's Personal Experiences of Public Sex Sites. Unpublished dissertation, Sociology Department, University of Colorado at Boulder.

Chng, C.L., Geliga-Vargas, J. (2000) "Ethnic Identity, Gay Identity, Sexual Sensation Seeking and HIV Risk Taking among Multiethnic Men Who Have Sex with Men." AIDS Education and Prevention. 12 (4): 326–339.

Clatts, M.C. (1999) Ethnographic Observations of Men Who have Sex with Men in Public: Toward an Ecology of Sexual Action. In W.L. Leap. (ed.) *Public* Sex/Gay Space (pp.141–155) New York: Columbia University Press.

Freitas, H.E. (1997) Has the Development of Protease Inhibitors Changed Sexual Behavior among Gay Men in Tucson, AZ? An Ethnographic Analysis of Three Focus Groups. Unpublished manuscript. Arizona Department of Health Services, November.

Freitas, H.E. (1996) The African American Men's Health Project: An Ethnographic Analysis of Sexual Decision-Making among Men between the Ages of 16-25. Unpublished manuscript. The Shanti Foundation.

Freitas, H.E. (1996b) Ethnographic Analysis of the Gay Men's Health Project: Targeting Gay Men Who Frequent Bars. Unpublished. manuscript. AIDS Prevention Collaboration.

Gross, M. (2003) "The Second Wave Will Drown Us." American Journal of Public Health, 93 (6): 872–881.

Hahn, R.A. (1999) *Anthropology and the Enhancement of Public Health Practices in Anthropology and Public Health.* Oxford: Oxford University Press. pp. 3–24.

Huebner, D., Formoso, D., Nemeroff, C., Proescholdbell, R.J. et al. (2001). Sexual Behaviors and HIV Prevention Service Use among Men Who Have Sex with Men: Final Report. Arizona State University Department of Psychology, June.

Humphreys, L. (1970) *Tearoom Trade: Impersonal Sex in Public Places*. Boston: Aldine Publishing Company.

Leap, W. (1999) *Public Sex/Gay Space.* New York: Columbia University Press.

Needle, R.H., Trotter, R.T., II, Singer, M. et al. (2003) "Rapid Assessment of the HIV/AIDS Crisis in Racial and Ethnic Minority Communities: an Approach for Timely Community Interventions." *American Journal of Public* Health 93 (6): 970–979.

Sieber, J. (2003) Laud Humphreys and the Tearoom Sex Study. http://www.missouri.edu/~philwb/Laud.html.

Southern Arizona AIDS Foundation (SAAF) (2003) Quarterly Report [of baseline data]. Prepared by Pima Prevention Partnership Planning and Evaluation Services. 10/15/03.

Weir, S.S., Pailman, C., Mahlalela, X. et al. (2003) "From People to Places: Focusing AIDS Prevention Efforts Where It Matters Most." *AIDS* 17 (6): 895–903.

Chapter 14

Conclusion: Assessing Primary, Secondary, and Future Benefits of Project RARE

Merrill Singer
Benjamin P. Bowser
Ernest Quimby

The Rapid Assessment, Response and Evaluation (RARE) project was born of a specific configuration of historic and social circumstances and events. It provides an insightful window to the American AIDS epidemic in the late twentieth and early twenty-first centuries. As a public health initiative, the RARE project is historically noteworthy on several grounds: 1) it adopted a rapid assessment and response strategy in the face of one of the most devastating diseases in human history (UNAIDS 2004); 2) it embraced often under-appreciated qualitative research methods to analyze a disease that has been measured, counted and quantified more than any previous human condition (Singer 2004); 3) it boldly attempted to unite the disconnected and conflicting research and service sectors into a collaborative, multifaceted team (Lamb et al. 1998); and 4) it honestly recognized that the U.S. AIDS epidemic of the early 1980s had "morphed" into a rather different epidemic by the late 1980s.

The new epidemic has become disproportionately a disease of people of color (including gay people of color) and a disease of poverty. Hence, issues of ethnic and racial social inequality, discrimination, and economic injustice have become critical determinants of the face of the epidemic (Friedman et al. 1987); and finally, 5) RARE responded to the fact that wherever AIDS has spread, the epidemic has taken on a strongly local character, affirming a notion embraced in RARE, that AIDS is a complex global pandemic composed of innumerable local epidemics, and that public health responses must be implemented accordingly (Mann et al. 1992). Each of these characteristics of RARE is discussed below and is evident in the earlier chapters of this book. This discussion is followed by the lessons learned from the RARE project, and the directions these lessons offer for prospective community responses to AIDS. As the prior chapters in this book suggest, RARE had its successes and its share of challenges in how a relatively small (narrowly funded) number of short-term projects can have a sustained and meaningful impact on local AIDS epidemics.

Bringing Rapid Methods Home

Rapid assessment methods were developed by U.S.-based researchers (Scrimshaw and Hurado 1987) in the late 1980s. For more than two decades now, rapid research methods have been used in diverse public health efforts in other countries around the world. In recent years, for example, the World Health Organization, Joint United Nations Programme on HIV/AIDS, Doctors Without Borders (Medicins sans frontiers), and the United Nations International Drug Control Programme have conducted AIDS-related rapid assessments. Its most effective use has been in resource-poor nations with limited budgets and small cadres of scientifically trained researchers (Needle et al. 2003; Weir et al. 2002), but rapid methods have also been used in HIV assessments in developed nations (Fenton et al. 2002). Ironically, rapid assessment has not been used broadly in the United States. Project RARE, in fact, represents the most extensive use of rapid assessment and response methods ever implemented in a U.S. public health program (Needle et al. 2000; Trotter et al. 2001).

For the most part, the RARE project has been implemented in the bleakest neighborhoods of impoverished cities among socially marginalized populations. The public health response to AIDS in these cities has been significantly challenged by shrinking local budgets, the wide availability of illicit drugs, racial/ethnic discrimination and tension, and the existence of multiple, competing health and social problems and significant health care disparities facing the poor, and communities of color. In such settings, the rapid, qualitative assessment approach has been particularly useful. Where this method has been implemented, field teams have found the project model so compelling that it has helped to drive each local project past looming barriers and dangerous pitfalls. The challenges include recruiting appropriate, usually part-time staff; finding ways to train staff quickly in how to collect behavioral and attitudinal data, a task that was brand new to most of the people staffing RARE projects around the country; the pressures of completing data collection, analyzing findings and formulating achievable recommendations in a timely fashion; and finding the means to widely disseminate and use the final reports to implement local change. Any one of these challenges might have doomed either local initiatives, or the project as a whole, to failure. In these cases they did not fail, however, because the methods used and the findings they produced helped to energize the community members who formed the local field teams in addition to the local project advisory committees and AIDS program administrators.

In a few cases, even the recognized benefits of carrying out the RARE project could not overcome pre-existing social conflicts and structural contradictions in local settings, thereby condemning the project to either very limited gains or outright failure. In one city, for example, turf wars among local decision-makers prevented the project from ever getting off the ground. In another city, internal conflicts drained the project of energy and prevented it from producing useful findings. In most instances, however, as represented by the chapters in this volume, RARE was on the whole successful, in no small measure because its methods, objectives, and benefits were readily grasped by those concerned with its implementation and with the utilization of findings.

Legitimating Qualitative Methods

RARE also represents a largely unique validation by the federal government of qualitative methods in health research since it has been implemented in U.S. cities and other settings from coast to coast, as well as a U.S.-controlled territory, the U.S. Virgin Islands. Historically, qualitative methods have been undervalued in epidemiology and public health. Seen as lacking objectivity, rigor and the replicability of quantitative methods, qualitative approaches often have been labeled "soft science," impressionistic, and overly dependant on the skills of the individual field worker. The AIDS epidemic, however, has played a significant role in revising conventional ways of thinking about research methods (Auerbach et al. 1994; Des Jarlais and Friedman 1998; Lambert et al. 1995; Parker and Ehrhardt 2001). Practitioners have found that quantitative methods have severe limitations in helping us to understand the AIDS epidemic. For example, one is not always certain about what the statistical relationships between behaviors actually mean. There is uncertainty about whether the words used in survey questions signify the same thing to respondents as they do to researchers. In addition, there are difficulties when studying at-risk populations whose actual social boundaries are unknown. In contrast, the epidemic has helped to reveal what qualitative methods are particularly good at, such as establishing social rapport with subjects in the study of private or illegal behaviors, locating hidden populations, discovering previously unknown behaviors, revealing cultural understandings, and revealing the impact of social and economic context on risk.

In the RARE project in Newark, New Jersey, for example, the field team found that commercial sex workers could be classified into two distinct types, that is those who worked for themselves and those who were "managed" by pimps, thereby helping them to understand how best to reach each group with the best HIV-prevention information. This was a discovery that most likely would not have been made through quantitative methods unless the survey or questionnaire happened to have focused on this issue. Newark field teams also identified senior citizens who were turning to commercial sex workers out of loneliness and boredom, and young whites from the suburbs who were spending increasingly more time using drugs on the streets of Newark, as being at high risk for HIV infection. By using observation techniques in its battery of qualitative methods, the Newark team realized they benefited from having "fresh eyes," that is, using field team leaders who were not familiar with the city and hence were not locked in to preconceived ideas about it.

As a result of his familiarity with RARE, the Surgeon General of the United States, David Satcher, significantly recognized how qualitative methods and ethnography have contributed to the achievement of critical public health goals by discussing this approach at several national conferences, including at the RARE national conference (via video hook-up). This is a level of recognition and legitimization that has long been denied these methods.

Uniting Research and Service

RARE can be seen as a way to overcome the common divide between research and service. Participation in RARE has required the "buy-in" of both researchers and the service community, but more important, it has required their collaboration. This work could not have succeeded without this alliance. Field teams consisted of experienced researchers and frontline community prevention workers. The Working Groups or community advisory committees in participating cities organized key local players in public health, community organizations, city government and other civic groups to use research findings to address local needs. In Chicago, for example, a by-product of this interaction was that community leaders were presented with strong research confirmation of the effectiveness of sterile syringe exchange in lowering HIV risk; this is an issue that is very contentious in some communities (Shaw and Singer 2003). At the same time, they saw firsthand how shrinking AIDS funding impacts prevention efforts, such as when they lost the ability to distribute sharp containers to shooting galleries to collect used and potentially infected needles, thereby taking them out of circulation. Since the advisory group had a hand in selecting target groups and zones, and helped to select the field team as well as to advise their efforts, team findings were more salient to decision-makers in pointing out clear directions for subsequent decision-making and action. Consequently, in cities like Hartford, Connecticut, the city health director immediately began efforts to implement changes in city contracts to insure late-night prevention measures (one of the project's local recommendations). Notably, as the local RARE project was winding down, these efforts were slowed when the city departments of social services and health were merged. Ultimately, however, late-night outreach was achieved. As this example shows, translating the findings of public health research into changes in policy is a difficult task. The "buy-in" component of RARE was specifically emphasized when designing the project to help overcome this potential barrier.

The New Epidemic

By supporting the RARE projects, the federal government expressed its awareness of a radical shift in the U.S. AIDS epidemic; it has expanded beyond white gay communities, to much larger heterosexual communities of color with hidden sub-groups of men who do not identify themselves as gay. In its earliest days, AIDS was called the "gay plague," as it appeared to strike primarily gay and bisexual men. By the time RARE was implemented, dramatic changes had occurred in the epidemic. Indigenous, community-level initiatives in gay communities around the country already led to a significant reduction in behaviors that facilitated the rapid diffusion of HIV among gay men (although that reduction has begun to turn around among younger gay/bisexual men). In addition, many gay men moved from big urban centers to smaller cities, towns and rural areas. But in low-income and impoverished communities of color, HIV infections were moving in the opposite direction. Massive numbers of new AIDS cases appeared with links to illicit drug use, and the mixing of commercial sex and drugs. While AIDS researchers had been aware of these trends for some time, community awareness and response lagged behind. By documenting local expressions of broader trends, RARE became most useful in bridging this gap between the leading edge of AIDS research and the movement of new knowledge about the epidemic from universities and research centers to frontline community decision-making and prevention efforts.

AIDS has come to thrive under conditions that Quimby, in Chapter 4, aptly refers to as minority "community destabilization," characterized by the flight of jobs, economic and social marginalization, and undermined cultural values. In the years before the initiation of the RARE project, 65% of the newly reported AIDS cases were occurring among African American and Latino adults. At the time, Latinos represented 13% and African Americans represented 12% of the total national population, yet they accounted for 20% and 45% respectively of all new AIDS cases. CDC's public announcement of these statistics in May 1998, led to the U.S. Congressional Black Caucus (CBC) to request that the Secretary of the Department of Health and Human Services, Donna Shalala, declare the HIV/AIDS epidemic in the African American community a "public health emergency." It was in response to this dramatic request that President Bill Clinton announced a comprehensive new initiative to improve the nation's effort to prevent the spread of AIDS in African American and Latino communities and to enhance the level of care provided to people of color living with the disease.

Finding the Community

RARE embodies the realization, often overlooked in our globalized world and in the midst of a pandemic, that on-the-ground AIDS is always a very local epidemic with distinctive local characteristics that must be understood if prevention efforts are to be effective. What works in Oakland, California, may be misguided for Baltimore, Maryland and counterproductive in Flagstaff, Arizona, or the Virgin Islands. The face of AIDS varies place-to-place across multiple dimensions. As the chapters of this book underline, there are a host of characteristics that give a unique shape to local AIDS epidemics: differences in ethnic composition, which populations are at greatest risk, primary routes of infection, local beliefs and practices, the organization of AIDS prevention efforts, and governmental structures. For example, in a city like Philadelphia, it was possible to identify a number of distinct "hot spots." There were small geographic zones with concentrated drug use and sex-related HIV risk; in contrast, the RARE team in Newark found that in that city, the notion of a narrow "geography of risk" was meaningless, since drug use was highly diffused.

In other words, from the beginning the RARE initiative took the concepts of locality and community seriously. The AIDS epidemic was viewed as far more than a biological disease. Rather, it was perceived as a complex set of interactions between a pathogenic agent and local populations within particular social and physical contexts. This included a range of local prevention responses (positive and negative) that developed in the face of the AIDS threat. Specifically, RARE understood local AIDS epidemics to be the product of an intersection between unique people, places and times. In this sense, RARE defines the commonly used, but rarely defined, concept of community as the social, locational and temporary intersection of behaviors, attitudes, and knowledge.

This concept of an epidemic as locally unique and shaped by native community factors was verified in each city. For instance, the time of day and the day of the month were particularly important in the expression of HIV-risk behaviors. As a consequence of the RARE projects' local focus, decisions were made at each site by local advisory groups to focus attention on their distinct combination of risk groups and neighborhoods. In Baltimore, for example, the target group was eighteen to twenty-four year olds living in two postal zones, while in Oakland the focus was on men who have sex with men, injection drug users, and commercial sex workers. Oakland included one group of women who rode the rapid transit system and engaged in commercial sex with customers in parking lots at the various stops along the route, and another group of HIV-positive women who did commercial sex in farm-worker camps on weekends. Other cities emphasized different groups who were believed to be at heightened risk for infection, defined by behavior, ethnicity, age, gender or other criteria. Without doubt, local politics or strong personalities on advisory teams influenced the local focus of RARE research. On the whole, however, advisory teams included a diverse mix of people who initially did not necessarily all agree about where to focus RARE data collection. Ultimately, discussion and compromise were used to narrow and define local priorities.

While a considerable amount of information is known about HIV—more, in fact than is known about any other virus that threatens humans—detailed knowledge about the local social environments of the epidemic is harder to come by. Systematically collected and ethnographically rich data on cultural patterns, ethnic relations, community-government interactions and popular attitudes about the disease are often lacking. Yet, as Mann et al. (1992:12) accurately stressed, "Information is liberating. It helps us to ask the right questions ..."

Often, AIDS prevention programs have been implemented around the country without a locally grounded, well-organized knowledge base to guide their efforts (Singer et al. 2005). RARE, in fact, began with the assumption that if AIDS was still spreading rapidly and widely in African American, Latino, and other ethnic minority communities, there may be identifiable gaps in the local knowledge and response systems. RARE sought to identify the moving edges of the epidemic by recognizing that there are populations, resources and numerous other differences between Chicago and West Palm Beach, and between Philadelphia and the Virgin Islands. These differences would be critical in shaping where, how and why (as well as among whom) the disease was spreading locally.

Of vital importance was the nature and structure of the local prevention effort in response to the epidemic. Was the local community fragmented and in conflict or unified and coordinated? Was the political structure sensitive to the needs of minority communities, and was there strong, stable leadership in the fight against the epidemic? Were there turf battles and resource squabbles among community organizations that prevented a unified and comprehensive response? Were there barriers to effectively reaching certain groups or parts of the city, or was prevention education not present where it was most needed? To illustrate this point, in Newark it was discovered that very high-risk regions of the city were systematically avoided by HIV-prevention efforts because it was assumed that they were too dangerous to enter. In such areas, in fact, the field team found numerous drug users interested in learning about treatment as well as sexually active individuals who were very happy to receive condoms. In Hartford, the field team found no evidence of late-night AIDS prevention efforts. This insured that many individuals who avoided the streets during the day and engaged in very high-risk behaviors late at night were completely unaware of local AIDS prevention efforts even though, during the day, there were multiple prevention programs in operation.

Recognizing that there were widely varying answers to the abovementioned questions in cities with HIV/AIDS epidemics, RARE intentionally grounded itself at each site in the local AIDS prevention and care effort, in on-the-ground community and political structures, and under the guidance of resident authorities, local advocates, and community-based programs. If the local community, ranging from the mayor (or equivalent) to frontline AIDS prevention workers and activists, did not endorse the RARE program, their application to conduct this research never went beyond preliminary discussions. Rather, it floundered early in the process and never got off the ground. It is important to point out that this was the case in a number of places around the country. Even if the program was implemented and completed in certain places, RARE faced disabling challenges if there was a lack of full support at any of several key political and community levels. Such was the case at the Washington, D.C., site.

By contrast, where buy-in was strong, field teams usually were quickly assembled; staffs were trained; and the suite of supported data collection and analytic methods were implemented with reasonable levels of success. These sites were able to develop a list of locally grounded recommendations that reflected immediate realities and needs. Even in cities that successfully implemented RARE, there were always challenges and hurdles to overcome. In Washington, D.C., field team members were recruited from the ranks of AIDS service providers and they did not switch comfortably to their new roles as data collectors. Despite these roadblocks and hurdles, field teams pressed on, fueled by a heartfelt desire to make a difference in the local AIDS epidemic. In the end, most were happy they did and felt that RARE had been a worthwhile endeavor in their fight against the epidemic.

Lessons from RARE

A number of things were learned from the RARE method that were not fully apparent at the outset, and certainly not clear from each site.

Locally Specific AIDS-Related Knowledge

RARE helped to uncover new knowledge of local HIV-risk patterns, community awareness, and attitudes, which assisted people in recognizing notable limitations within existing AIDS prevention and service delivery. As the previous chapters have described, in almost all RARE cities, key information of populations at risk, locations of risk, attitudes of people at greatest risk, consumer ideas for enhanced intervention, barriers to risk reduction, and related topics was added by RARE to the local knowledge base. This new knowledge was critical in shaping subsequent AIDS prevention and service efforts. In Miami, for example, identification of "*makrel*" houses of prostitution used by Haitians had been "invisible" to outsiders who were not part of local sex networks prior to RARE. With this new knowledge, HIV-prevention efforts could be targeted to these high-risk sites. In Palm Beach County, Florida, the field team found inadequate access to HIV-preventive and patient care services in the areas the RARE project targeted for data collection. Moreover, they found that some community prevention workers were quite critical of the quality of local HIV patient care services. Some provider institutions were not welcoming toward patients from high-risk areas. Findings like these helped to mobilize efforts for change in many RARE cities. Nowhere were the changes stimulated by RARE sufficient to stem the epidemic, but RARE did help to make improvements in local services.

Pressing Intervention Needs

The RARE initiative discovered specific local, as well as cross-site, intervention needs. For example, a number of RARE projects found that there was a serious gap between the hours during which street prevention efforts occurred and the peak hours of AIDS risk. RARE revealed on a national scale that there was a critical need for late-night prevention education on HIV risks and services. At local sites, numerous site-specific intervention needs were also identified, and communicated in the form of specific recommendations to public health officials. As a result, in many—but not all RARE cities—changes were made in local policies and programs. The implementation of late-night outreach to high-risk individuals in Oakland is an example of how RARE project recommendations led to local changes in AIDS prevention efforts. In Hartford, RARE provided information that was used to help restore state funding to syringe exchange programs. Similar changes occurred in other RARE cities.

Educating Decision-Makers

Having authority in a local public health system, or being the head of a community-based organization, does not guarantee extensive AIDS-related knowledge grounded in local community beliefs and practices. As noted in the previous chapters, in several sites RARE was found to contribute to the improvement of the knowledge base of local decision-makers concerning HIV-risk patterns and community knowledge deficits. This new level of understanding was commonly expressed at the final, community-wide meetings of RARE projects and in the final reports produced at each site. As a result, in many cities public health and other officials expressed appreciation for the information they learned from the RARE initiative. In some cases—such as the information provided by the Washington, D.C., project on the way AIDS stigma served as a barrier to seeking treatment—was not well received by local officials because it came with a recommendation to send mobile vans into communities for testing and counseling.

Micro-Environments

In a number of cities, the local RARE project led to the discovery of significant differences in risk at the block level within seemingly uniform neighborhoods. In Chicago, for example, neighborhoods like the Far West Side, Humboldt Park and Atgeld Gardens had noticeably different resources, at-risk populations, and risk configurations requiring differing prevention responses. Field team leaders in Philadelphia labeled especially risky areas "hot spots," a concept that was subsequently adopted by a number of other RARE sites. In several RARE cities, these geographically circumscribed but socially fluid risk zones were geo-epicenters driving the local HIV epidemic. In short, a key lesson from RARE was that risk must be assessed more deeply than at the city level. It is important to recognize that cities, or even towns, are composed of diverse micro-environments, which range in their level of AIDS risk behavior. Targeting the highest risk areas, it follows, is a strategic approach to AIDS prevention (Des Jarlais, Padian, Winkelstein 1994).

In addition to the primary gains discussed above, there were other benefits of the RARE initiative that were as important as the primary contributions to local prevention and intervention efforts. A number of these secondary benefits of RARE are discussed below.

Skill Transfer

RARE was able to make a recognizable contribution to the transfer of new skills and the development of an infrastructure for the rapid assessment of other unmet prevention needs in local settings. While the focus of RARE was on the AIDS epidemic, the methods skill set it provided helped cities to adapt the RARE model to address other local public health issues like teen pregnancy or children's nutrition. In Hartford, for example, members of the RARE team worked with the Connecticut Department of Public Health to implement a rapid assessment of teen pregnancy among Latinas. During the final meeting with the project's advisory group, a field team member in Detroit stated, "The team process help[ed] to build the skill sets of community outreach workers and educators." In addition, the project helped to disperse existing skills within the community. Another field team member in Detroit reported, "We trained each other, we supported each other, we relied on skills we had before the process began" (Singer 2000). In other words, RARE brought in outside professional trainers who introduced research skills to local service providers. It also facilitated skills-sharing among prevention workers who previously might not have had opportunities to work together.

AIDS Prevention Planning

The RARE model provides a clearly articulated and easily adopted methodology for the development of evidence-based AIDS prevention planning which has been woefully lacking in many cities. While the community prevention model from the Centers for Disease Control and Prevention has successfully helped to implement local planning groups at the state or local level throughout the country, and while these entities are expected to use an evidence-based approach to set prevention priorities, the capacity for new data collection is not always available. In a number of sites, the RARE model has found utility in meeting this critical need.

Generally, across sites, RARE project staff observed that the RARE methodology offered an important new approach for empirically grounded HIV prevention. In particular, this method was valued by people working on RARE projects because it rapidly revealed previously unknown places, times, and social patterns that put people at risk for HIV, made it possible to translate this new knowledge immediately into useable concepts, and expedited the transfer of these formulations directly to decision-makers and service providers in the form of concrete public health recommendations. As a city health official in Philadelphia noted during a project meeting, "The strengths and benefits of the field approach were the ability to be able to gather information on a vulnerable population which is extremely difficult to gather through any other method than the one used. The teams' mobility, wide geographic scope, and schedule of hours (around the clock) ensured that the information gathered through informant interviews was reflective of the realities, perceptions and needs of the study's target population" (Singer 2000). At the same time it should be noted that when RARE findings and recommendations are subsequently ignored in local AIDS planning efforts, considerable frustration can result. This can be seen, for example, in the failure of the federal government to respond to significant findings on the effectiveness of syringe exchange in lowering HIV risk among drug users which has happened repeatedly during the AIDS epidemic. The common time delays between the completion of RARE projects and changes in local prevention planning also can contribute to this unfortunate turn of events.

Identification of Barriers to Change

The RARE model offers a useful approach for pinpointing institutional barriers to the dissemination of consistent public health messages, roadblocks to service access and utilization, and shortcomings in service quality and resources. In Miami and Chicago, for example, RARE data collection revealed that local police detain people for carrying condoms on the grounds that condom possession suggests involvement in prostitution. Of course, condom promotion has been a central element in many AIDS prevention campaigns, worldwide. Institutional barriers to condom use as a public health measure constitute a dangerous health policy (Arachu and Singer 2004). Similarly, the Oakland site detected that police use syringe exchange sites to investigate drug users and to confiscate their used and newly exchanged sterile needles, thereby diminishing the effectiveness of the syringe exchange program. In Palm Beach, the project encountered that Haitians and Guatemalans were afraid to go the Department of Health's main HIV clinic because the U.S. Immigration and Naturalization Services (INS) office was located in the same building.

In other cities, like Baltimore, attitudes held in the community constituted barriers to AIDS prevention. Many youth in Baltimore see HIV testing as risky. If diagnosed as being HIV-positive, they reasoned, they would lose social support, love and acceptance. In addition, it was discovered that people in Baltimore choose to engage in unprotected sexual intercourse because it reduces exposure to another risk, namely social isolation. In short, a network of social barriers, including "AIDS stigma," the willingness to engage in sex without a condom in order to achieve other desired ends, and considerable misinformation about the disease and the nature of services, push youth in Baltimore to avoid using HIV/AIDS prevention services altogether. These were significant challenges to service providers which have to be overcome to combat the epidemic.

A very different set of challenges exists in Tucson. A significant barrier was presented by the large number of sites local MSMs use to pick up other men (more than sixty-five in Tucson alone, plus various other sites in nearby towns, as well as in Mexico and California). A major problem for local AIDS prevention efforts in Tucson is how best to make an impact under such a diversity of risk-sites.

Re-Invigoration

AIDS prevention is stressful. Being involved in this work longterm means health workers and researchers alike will endure the illness and deaths of some people they have assisted and come to care for over time. Consequently, the potential for "burn out" is great, which RARE field teams found among AIDS workers. One of the unintended impacts of the RARE initiative was that participation in the project helped to produce a significant level of renewed enthusiasm among frontline prevention workers. In a number of "RARE cities" the field staff felt empowered with new skills they could use in making their AIDS efforts more effective. In some places, they were able to become advocates for the changes suggested by the RARE study. At the same time, the RARE unification of researchers, decision-makers, and field team members in a common effort led to frontline staff feeling that their voices were being heard "at the top" for the first time.

A Final Key Finding of the RARE Initiative

RARE recommendations were born out of a sense of urgency and a need to act decisively to address the march of AIDS in communities of color in the U.S. In the communities in which it was implemented, RARE helped to identify the frontline of the epidemic: people and places where risks existed and disease was occurring. Pragmatic recommendations were made about what could be done to fight the epidemic. Local public health departments were involved; federal officials were involved; local community-based agencies and community members were involved. RARE provided timely information to the right people. Everything was in place for decisive action to reduce, if not stop, the spread of AIDS in poor communities of color. Most RARE recommendations at the majority of participating sites were taken into advisement and put before planning and other committees. Five years later, the list of implemented recommendations is far shorter than project participants would have hoped for. Instead, as has been the case too often during the AIDS epidemic, it has been business as usual. In all of the RARE sites, public health authorities complained that they needed more federal funding to fully implement the RARE recommendations. The federal response in return was that local authorities were already given Congressional Black Caucus funding and other funding for AIDS prevention through their state governments; it was up to local authorities to act.

Business as usual in the face of a potential health crisis is nothing new. We continue to witness public health immobility with regard to diabetes, drug abuse, obesity, hepatitis C, and further efforts against smoking. Immobility in response to seriously contagious diseases among African Americans has a long history. In fact, no contagious disease that has been primarily concentrated in African American communities has ever been aggressively addressed by federal and State authorities. This was the case for yellow fever, tuberculosis, and syphilis early in the past century. It required an African American, community-based health movement at the turn of the last century to effectively address these diseases. It is this past and continuing history that has led to current racial disparities in virtually every health indicator (Budrys 2003; Fiscella 2002; McBride 1991). African Americans consistently have had higher infant mortality, higher age-adjusted mortality, higher rates for almost every infectious disease, higher rates of drug abuse, poorer health care, and have received less aggressive medical treatment when it is warranted (Williams 1995; Lillie-Blanton 1996). So far, it has been no different with the AIDS epidemic, which now can be added to this infamous list. This, however, was not a failure of the RARE methodology, or of the commitment of local field teams, or of the effort to build research/community partnership as a core element in RARE.

Conclusion

Overall, it was found that cities involved in the RARE project, despite their having quite different human and fiscal resources and public health structures, were able to: 1) successfully adopt the RARE rapid ethnographic methodology; 2) collect new information about HIV-risk times, places and populations, including a wide range of discoveries about how the epidemic was being spread locally and limitations on existing HIV-prevention approaches; and 3) formulated specific useful recommendations for implementation. A key strength of RARE as a qualitative methodology influenced by the ethnographic model of research is that it allows healthcare providers and policy makers to hear the insider perspective from individuals in their own city or locale. These are the people who are actually engaged in high-risk behavior that make their own indigenous recommendations for the types of changes they believe would lower HIV risk.

As a result of RARE findings and recommendations, some changes have been made in local AIDS efforts. Here are but three examples: 1) in Newark, training of AIDS prevention staff has been enhanced while outreach has been adopted as a core prevention strategy; 2) in Hartford, late-night syringe exchange has been implemented and the city Department of Health and Human Services is now mandating late-night prevention services. A citywide community effort is also underway to implement a late-night, drop-in center for individuals at risk of infection; and 3) in Chicago, RARE findings were used to successfully advocate for increased funding for the Department of Health's Division of STD/HIV/AIDS for HIV/AIDS prevention and care programs.

In several sites around the country, RARE has had some identifiable impacts on local HIV-prevention discourse, planning, and programming. Progress is greater in some cities than others, and some recommendations have been more easily adopted than others. Implementing the late-night, drop-in center in Hartford, for example, has faced a local barrier (e.g., former church space that was to be made available for the center by a community organization did not meet city code requirements because of a fire). Miami was able to implement a number of RARE recommendations because local funding was made available by the city for this purpose. The same was true in Oakland, which developed local funding for the RARE-recommended night outreach program targeting HIV risk—the U.S. Office of AIDS was provided funds to recruit and test late-night, high-risk takers. Other cities have not been able to achieve as much, more often because of fiscal constraints. In a number of cities, like Philadelphia, Miami, and Hartford, RARE findings have been incorporated into local planning efforts, grant-writing initiatives, and funding allocation decisions; these are all significant achievements for the RARE initiative.

This is not to say, as we have noted above, that the RARE project did not encounter significant problems and challenges. Some of these were site-specific and reflected local issues, tensions, and political barriers. Others were inherent in the RARE structure and funding levels. Sometimes, field staff members were late in being paid, other times necessary equipment (e.g., transcription machines) was not available. Field team leaders in several cities complained that they were not given a role in the selection of field team members, a process that may have been completed before the leader was hired. As a result, field teams sometimes included members who the team leaders would not have selected to be on the team. Field teams often were composed of individuals who previously had been engaged in service delivery, so members who had little or no experience with conducting research tended to blur research and service together. In some cases, the training of field team members proved to be inadequate and attrition among field teams (who were, by design, part-timers on the project) was a problem. In other cases, the final RARE report was not well-received, because its findings suggested shortcomings of previous efforts or was viewed as introducing a competing agenda with an existing prevention plan. In a few cases, some community leaders complained that there was nothing new in the RARE findings. In other instances, such as the Washington, D.C., RARE site, the colonial structure under which the city is governed by Congress and the institutional inertia that exists insured that project findings and recommendations would be largely ignored.

Given the small number of staff working on the project in the Washington headquarters, communication with the central leadership was sometimes difficult. At some sites there was resistance to adhering to the RARE project model. In some cases, local public health bureaucracy, inefficiency, and the lack of anything that resembled adequate funding stymied or completely undercut the impact of RARE. In other instances, however, problems in the local public health structure helped to facilitate the project. Despite these difficulties, many of which caused varying degrees of frustration at local sites or among national administrators of the project, RARE's shorter-term successes ultimately far outnumbered the project's shortcomings, and RARE had an immediate positive impact on AIDS and other public health work at many (but not all) local sites where it was implemented around the country.

As a consequence, the RARE model has been adopted (and adapted) for use by the Human Resources Services Administration (HRSA) in the study of why many people with HIV/AIDS (from various ethnic groups or at-risk populations) do not get into care services or drop out of them early. As defined by the U.S. Department of Health and Human Services, "care" means the receipt of primary medical care for HIV disease that is consistent with U.S. Public Health Service Treatment Guidelines. Such care must include access to antiretroviral and other drug therapies, including prophylaxis and treatment of opportunistic infections, and combination antiretroviral therapies. Individuals are considered "in care" if they access HIV-related support services such as case management, transportation assistance, or personal counselling but do not receive primary medical care. This study is being implemented in three cities around the country, with potential for broader implementation in future years.

A broader question concerns the longer-term impact of RARE. Short-term successes need not mount up to longer-term impact on the AIDS epidemic in any local setting and may say nothing of having any effect at the national level. Further, each RARE project was narrowly funded and received less than a year of federal support. Staffs on the projects were part-time, and most had no prior research experience. Project research directors commonly did not meet their staff until just before the beginning of staff training. Moreover, the projects were usually implemented in urban areas with significant fiscal problems, multiple pressing health and social issues, and entrenched bureaucracies with existing agendas. Ultimately, the longer-term impact of any of the RARE projects was determined by the stability and commitment of the organizational entity and local actors who implemented the project. When implemented by an organization with stable leadership and a commitment to evidence-based public health programming, RARE findings and recommendations remain on the agenda of local public health decision-making years after the formal project ends. Where there is lacking a strong local advocacy for the implementation of RARE recommendations, the longer-term local impact of RARE is very limited, at best.

At the national level, the adoption of the RARE model by HRSA points to its future direction. The methodology continues to have considerable value for ongoing AIDS prevention, and additional sites have implemented the model since the completion of the cases described in this book. The RARE approach holds considerable potential as a community-based, scientifically sound strategy for timely public health information gathering and decision making across the full breadth of pressing health issues of concern among low income communities of color. The value of the RARE model for achieving needed change is evident in light of the growing recognition that health disparity is widespread and consequential, and populations like those described in this book are denied equal access to quality health care. Nonetheless, if there is one enduring lesson of the RARE project it is this: the RARE approach is only of value if there is an authentic commitment to doing all that is possible to stop the AIDS epidemic, especially for the hardest hit groups and in the most troubled communities. RARE findings and recommendations—like all public health research—are only of value if they are used to guide policy and programs. Left on a shelf to gather dust along with previous reports, assessments, and evaluations, means RARE reports are not worth the trees used to make the paper they are printed on. But when employed to change the environment of risk and care, they are priceless.

References

Auerbach, J., Wypijewska, C., and Brodie, H. (1994) *AIDS and Behavior*. Washington: National Academy Press.

Budrys, Grace (2003) *Unequal Health: How Inequality Contributes to Health or Illness*. Roman & Lanham, MD: Littlefield Publishers.

Castro, Arachu, Singer, M. (2004) *Unhealthy Health Policy: A Critical Anthropological Examination*. Walnut Creek, CA: Altamira Press.

Des Jarlais, D., Padian, N., Winkelstein, W. (1994) "Targeted HIV-prevention Programs." New England Journal of Medicine. 331 (21): 1451–1453.

Des Jarlais, Don, Friedman, S. (1998) "Fifteen Years of Research on Preventing HIV Infection among Injecting Drug Users: What We Have Learned, What We Have not Learned, What We Have Done, What We Have not Done." Public Health Reports 113 (Supplement 1): 182–188.

Fenton, K., Chinouya, M., Davidson, O., and Copras, A. (2002) "HIV testing and High Risk Sexual Behavior among London's Migrant Communities: A Participatory Research Study." Sexually Transmitted Diseases 78 (4): 241–245.

Fiscella, K., Franks, P., Doescher, M., Saver, B. (2002) "Disparities in Health Care by Race, Ethnicity, and Language among the Insured: findings from a National Study." Medical Care 40 (1): 52–59.

Friedman, Samuel, Sotheran, J., Abdul-Quader, A. et al. (1987). "The AIDS Epidemic among Blacks and Hispanics." *The Milbank Quarterly* 65 (2): 455–499.

Lamb, Sara, Greenlick, M.R., McCarty, D. (eds.) (1998) *Bridging the Gap Between Practice and Research: Forging Partnerships with Community-Based Drug and Alcohol Treatment*. Washington: National Academy Press.

Lambert, Elizabeth, Ashery, R., and Needle, R., (eds.) (1995) *Qualitative Methods in Drug Abuse and HIV Research.* (pp. 231–257). National Institute on Drug Abuse Research Monographs No. 157. Washington: National Institute on Drug Abuse.

Lillie-Blanton (1996) "Race/ethnicity, the social environment, and health." *Social* Science and Medicine 43: 83–92.

Mann, Jonathan, Tarantola, D., Netter, T. (1992) *AIDS in the World: A Global Report.* Cambridge, MA: Harvard University Press.

McBride, David (1991) *From TB to AIDS: Epidemics among Urban Blacks Since 1900.* Albany: State University of New York Press.

Needle, Richard, Trotter, R., II, Goosby, E., Bates, C.,Von Zinkernagel, D. (2000). "Methodologically Sound Rapid Assessment and Response: Providing Timely Data for Policy Development on Drug Use Interventions." *International* Journal of Drug Policy 11: 19–23.

Needle, Richard, Trotter, T., II, Singer, M., et al. (2003) "Rapid Assessment of HIV/AIDS Crisis in Racial and Ethnic Minority Communities: An Approach for Timely Community Interventions." *American Journal of Public* Health 93 (6): 970–979.

Parker, Richard, Ehrhardt, A. (2001) "Through an Ethnographic Lens: Ethnographic Methods, Comparative Analysis and HIV/AIDS Research." *AIDS* and Behavior 5 (2): 105–114.

Scrimshaw, Susan, Hutado, E. (1987) *Rapid Assessment Procedures for Nutrition and Primary Health Care: Anthropological Approaches to Improving Programme Effectiveness.* Los Angeles: University of California Latin American Center Publications.

Singer, Merrill (2000). *Interim Evaluator's Report: Rapid Assessment, Response, and Evaluation Project (RARE): Philadelphia, Detroit and Miami.* Washington: Office of HIV/AIDS Policy, the Department of Health and Human Services.

Singer, Merrill (2004). An Epidemic by the Numbers: Categorizing, Counting and Constructing AIDS. Presented at The Political and Symbolic Implications of Quantification Conference. Brown University, Providence, RI.

Shaw, S., Singer, M. (2003). "Communities in Conflict: The Struggle for AIDS Prevention." Practicing Anthropology 25 (3): 12–15.

Singer, Merrill, Stopka, T., Shaw, S., et al. (2005) "Lessons from the Field: From Research to Application in the Fight Against AIDS among Injection Drug Users in Three New England Cities." *Human Organization* 64 (2):179–191.

Trotter, Robert, Needle, R., Goosby, E., et al. (2001) "A Methodological Model for Rapid Assessment, Response, and Evaluation: The RARE Program in Public Health." Field Methods 13 (2): 137–159.

UNAIDS (2004) *Report on the Global AIDS Epidemic.* Geneva: The United Nations.

Weir, S., Moroni, C., Coetzee, N., et al. (2002) "A Pilot Study of a Rapid Assessment Method to Identify Places for AIDS Prevention in Cape Town, South Africa." Sexually Transmitted Diseases 78 (Supplement 1): 106–113.

Williams, David. R., Collins, C. (1995) "U.S. Socioeconomic and Racial Differences in Health: Patterns and Explanations." *Annual Review of Sociology* 21: 349–386.

Index

About the Contributors

Benjamin P. Bowser, Ph.D. is professor and chair of sociology and social services at California State University, East Bay, in Hayward, California, where he was outstanding professor of 1996. He was visiting professor at The University of Paris (Sorbonne) in 2005, has served on two Institution of Medicine study panels focused on drug abuse and HIV prevention, and is on the advisory board of the University of California Universitywide AIDS Research Program. He is a board member of the Glide Foundation (San Francisco) and research advisor for the California Prevention Education Program (Cal-Pep), and U.S. associate editor of *Sage Race Relations Abstracts* (London). Among other works, Professor Bowser is lead editor of *Preventing AIDS: Community-Science Collaboration* (2004), The Social Dimensions of AIDS: A Sociology of the AIDS Epidemic (*International Journal of Sociology and Social Policy* (2002), *Against the Odds: Scholars Who Challenged Race in the Twentieth Century* (2002), *and Impacts of Racism on White Americans* (1996).

Alix Conde is a research associate at the National Development and Research Institutes (NDRI) in New York City. With a B.A. degree in anthropology from Berkeley, he has a long history of research on HIV/AIDS, drugs and the Haitian diaspora. He is currently working on a CDC-funded project on drug injectors in New York City.

Ric Curtis, Ph.D. is the chair of the anthropology department at the John Jay College of Criminal Justice, and has more than twenty-five years of experience conducting ethnographic research in New York City neighborhoods. He has written numerous publications on drugs, gangs, and HIV/AIDS. He also has a record of activism in New York City, especially in the area of harm reduction, and serves on the boards of directors of several local social service organizations, including Family Services Network and the After Hours Project in Brooklyn, and CitiWide Harm Reduction in the Bronx.

Karen Dodge, Ph.D. works in the Palm Beach County Health Department and in the department of epidemiology and public health at the University of Miami Miller School of Medicine. Her areas of interest are substance abuse; HIV/AIDS; and broad-based community health. She is a consultant for CDC and HRSA and a grant review panelist for NIH: Community Health. Her research areas are methodologies incorporating qualitative and quantitative techniques, path analyses, repeat measures of ANOVA and regression technique.

Julie M. Eiserman was the field coordinator of RARE Hartford for the Hispanic Health Council in Hartford, Connecticut. She received her M.A. in medical anthropology from Case Western Reserve University in 1998. She has spent the last 9+ years conducting both qualitative and quantitative research in applied, non-profit, clinical and academic settings. She has conducted research in the areas of Alzheimer's disease, alcohol abuse, club drug use, sexually transmitted diseases, injection drug use, mental health treatment for dual diagnosed Latinos, condom use, and pharmaceutical drug prescribing and use, among other things. Currently, she conducts market research at Millward Brown in Fairfield, CT.

Barbara Feeney is in the doctoral program at Florida State University and has served as health planner for the Treasure Coast Health Council since 2000. Since 1998, she have conducted local, regional, state, and federal research and planning projects for twenty-five counties throughout the state of Florida. These projects include work on high-crime rate communities, People with Disabilities, disaster planning, migrant workers, HIV/AIDS, tobacco prevention, diabetes, emergency services, and rural health care as well as district health plans and strategic planning initiatives. In addition to health planning, she has more than twenty-five years experience in teaching and social work with children and their families.

Halley Freitas has worked in research program design and evaluation of marginalized populations over the last fifteen years. Trained first as an anthropologist, she integrates a comprehensive blend of qualitative and quantitative research methods to all of her work. For ten years, she consulted for Pima County's various non-profit AIDS prevention organizations in cutting edge research and subsequent program development for high risk populations. Because these diverse programs were developed in cooperation with the targeted population, these program interventions continue to be relevant and still exist today.

Barbara Hill, Ph.D. has fourteen years of experience working for local county health departments. She recently accepted a position as the community research and data coordinator for Healthy House, a non-profit community organization in Merced, CA. She holds a doctoral in public health. She has work experience in several areas within health department systems such as communicable disease control, epidemiology, maternal and child health, health education and administration. She also teaches and consults. Her current focus is in improving community health through building collaborations between public institutions and non-profit community organizations in communities, and through community-based participation and evaluation.

Maria Irizarry is currently the Senior Director of Grants & Community Health for Catholic Health and Human Services, an inner city multi-hospital and community based system serving Newark and the four surrounding counties. Prior to her current position, Maria served as the AIDS director for the City of Newark in the Newark Department of Health & Human Services. She is the vice chair of the Newark Eligible Metropolitan Area Health Services Planning Council, and an executive member of the N.J Governor's Council for

HIV/AIDS. She also serves on the board of directors of the CAEAR Coalition a National Advocacy group that works on behalf of communities advocating emergency AIDS relief.

Paul LaKosky is a Ph.D. candidate in the department of anthropology at the University of Illinois at Chicago. His academic interests include medical anthropology, risk theory, systems theory and HIV. In addition, he is the Director of Capacity Building, Training, and Technical Assistance for the Division of STD/HIV/AIDS Public Policy and Programs at the Chicago Department of Public Health.

Louis Herns Marcelin, Ph.D. is director of research at the Family and Youth Community Research Center, Inc. of which is a co-founder. He is a research faculty member at University of Miami and the principal investigator for the Haitian Adolescent Study at the Department of Anthropology and Department of epidemiology and public health. He recently completed a large-scale NIDA funded study of youth gangs and delinquency in Miami-Dade, Florida. He is also conducting research both in Brazil and Haiti on family, kinship, and politics as well as on uses of political violence in Haiti.

Floyd Meeks has worked in various capacities in HIV since 1988. He has done HIV counseling and testing, HIV health education, worked at the state level monitoring Prevention and Ryan White Title II grants, and is currently the Program Coordinator for HIV Prevention and Surveillance for the Pima County Health Department.

Agatha Nelson, Ph.D. recently retired as associate professor of Psychology in the social sciences division of the University of the Virgin Islands (St. Thomas campus). She earned a B.A. in cultural anthropology as well as an M.A. in developmental psychology from Hunter College of the City University of New York. She also earned an M.A. in education (Tests and Measurements) from New York University. Her Ph.D. and M.Phil. are from the City University Graduate Center (CUNY). Over the past fifteen years Dr. Nelson has participated in several studies dealing with HIV/AIDS. She is a charter member of the Association of Virgin Islands Psychologists (AVIP) and a lifetime member of the Caribbean Studies Association (CSA). She has also been a member of the American Psychological Association and the Association of Black Psychologists.

Lawrence Ouellet, Ph.D. is a research associate professor in the Division of Epidemiology and Biostatistics, University of Illinois at Chicago, School of Public Health. He directs UIC's Community Outreach Intervention Projects (COIP), which since 1986 has conducted research and provided services focused on preventing HIV and other infectious diseases among substance users. He is a sociologist and ethnographer, and the principal investigator on several projects, including NIDA-funded studies examining the drug-related sexual diffusion of HIV infection from behaviorally high-risk to lower risk populations and transitions into drug injection by young people who sniff heroin. His publications include studies of sex-for-crack exchanges, the social organization of 'shooting galleries', incident HIV infection among sex partners of injection drug users, and the nomenclature associated with crack cocaine and its impact on risk reduction messages.

J. Bryan Page, Ph.D. is professor and chair, department of anthropology, University of Miami. Dr. Page studies the consumption of drugs and risk for HIV among marginalized populations in Miami-Dade. He is also an adjunct professor at the department of sociology, University of Miami.

Dr. Arvilla Payne-Jackson, Ph.D. is a full professor at Howard University. She received her doctorate from the University of Pennsylvania. Her primary areas of research are in the fields of medical anthropology, sociolinguistics, ethnographic evaluation and service learning. She has conducted fieldwork in the United States, the Caribbean, Latin America and Africa. Dr. Payne-Jackson has published three books, one monograph and numerous articles, several of which have been co-authored with students. She was executive producer of a full-length documentary on African American Folk medicine. In addition to being lead ethnographer with Dr. Quimby on the RARE project, she has done consulting work for the Office of National Drug Control Policy; Center for Substance Abuse; Early Head Start; Comprehensive Child Development Project; Innovation Center/4H-Youth-Adult Service Learning Projects; Department of Labor: Youth Opportunities Initiative; Marshall Heights Community Development Organization: Fighting Back Initiative; and Jamaica Blue Cross, among others.

Ernest Quimby, Ph.D. is associate professor of sociology at Howard University. His major research interests are cultural competence, HIV/AIDS, mental health services, urban community development, substance abuse, and juvenile/criminal justice issues. His professional work involves the evaluation of vocational services and supported employment for adults with severe and persistent mental illness, and the assessment of cultural competence of evidence-based practices for mental health services. He has been a researcher on projects funded by the National Institute on Drug Abuse, National Institute on Alcoholism and Alcohol Abuse, National Institute of Mental Health, and Substance Abuse and Mental Health Services Administration. He served as a lead ethnographer for the RARE projects in the District of Columbia and Baltimore, MD. He is a member of the African American Researchers and Scholars Group, an advisory body to NIDA. He also chairs the HIV/AIDS Coalition of the African American Health Program sponsored by the Health and Human Services Department of Montgomery County, MD.

Merrill Singer, Ph.D. is director of research at the Hispanic Health Council's Center for Community Health Research and helped to design the RARE evaluation program as a national RARE evaluator. He also directed the Hartford RARE project. Dr. Singer is the author, co-author, or editor of fifteen books and has authored over 170 health and social science articles. A medical anthropologist with a primary focus on health disparities in the U.S., he is a recent recipient of both the Society for the Anthropology of North America Prize for Distinguished Achievement in the Critical Study of North America and the Society for Medical Anthropology's Practicing Anthropology Award.

Patricia Rhymer Todman, Ph.D. is professor of psychology and coordinator of the psychology program at the University of the Virgin Islands. Since 1988 she has maintained a part-time clinical practice in psychology in the British Virgin Islands and U.S. Virgin Islands. Dr. Todman received her Ph.D. in clinical/ community psychology from the University of California at Berkeley in 1987, and her undergraduate baccalaureate degree in psychology and social relations in 1976 from Harvard University. Dr. Todman is Founding President and Member of the Association of (U.S.) Virgin Islands Psychologists, Member of the (U.S.) Virgin Islands Board of Psychology Examiners and the BVI Allied Health Professionals Council. She also engages in research on children's status indicators as well as consultation and evaluation of health service delivery programs.

Robert T. Trotter, II, Ph.D. is an Arizona Regent's Professor in Anthropology. He is a medical anthropologist with twenty-five years of experience in cross-cultural health issues ranging from traditional healing in Mexican American communities to alcohol, drug abuse and HIV prevention and intervention programs for minority groups in the U.S. and in international settings. Dr. Trotter has more than 100 publications in scientific books and journals and has conducted research and policy studies for the National Institutes of Health, World Health Organization, and the Centers for Disease Control and Prevention. He has a commitment to exploring new ethnographic research methods, research design, computer assisted ethnography, and international training in rapid ethnographic assessment, including the RARE and I-RARE programs for DHHS and CDC. His other interest is the area of research ethics. His publications include books and articles on Mexican American traditional healing, cross-cultural alcohol and drug studies, migrant farm worker health and education, prevention and intervention studies on HIV/AIDS, alcohol, and drug use, cross-cultural applicability research on disabilities and the international classification of disease. He is also an author on a pending patent "System and Model for Performance Value Based Collaborative Relationships" (GP-303794: 845OR-66).

Elijah Ward, Ph.D. is a postdoctoral research fellow in the Illinois Public Health Research Fellowship Program at the University of Illinois at Chicago.

His doctorate was in sociology at Northwestern University. His dissertation was based on his ethnography of a hospice, entitled, "Boundaries in the Heart: The Sociology of Distance and Intimacy in Hospice Work." Elijah has conducted research across several projects on the socio-behavioral dimensions of HIV. His current work explores social dimensions of the spiritual practices of devotional communities.

Tina Wolf is a Ph.D. student in criminal justice at John Jay College of Criminal Justice. She is completing a study of drug dealers in Rochester, NY, and is currently working on an NIJ-funded study of prostituting teenagers in New York City.